This is ME Doing LIFE

MY JOURNEY OF SELF-CARE AND SELF-REFLECTION

By Victoria McCune

Inspired Forever Book Publishing
Dallas, Texas

This is Me Doing Life: My Journey of Self-Care and Self-Reflection

Copyright © 2019 Victoria McCune

All rights reserved, including the right of reproduction in whole or in part in any form without prior written permission, except in the case of brief quotations embodied in critical reviews and certain other noncommercial uses permitted by copyright law.

Inspired Forever Book Publishing™
"Words With Lasting Impact"
Dallas, Texas
(888) 403-2727

Printed in the United States of America

Library of Congress Control Number: 2019940949
Softcover ISBN-13: 978-1-948903-13-4

Disclaimer: This is written as a true-to-life work of fiction. Names, characters, businesses, places, events, locales, and incidents may have been changed in order to protect certain identities as a matter of privacy.

DEDICATION

To all my fellow caregivers: May the work you do every day never go unnoticed, and may we stand together to provide support to one another. Let us not forget we are humans ourselves and have valid hopes and dreams that don't deserve to be placed on a back burner.

PREFACE

I was inspired to write this book in the hope that it will encourage others to tell their stories. We each have a past; whether our pasts are good or bad, we each have one. I have never had any formal sit-down therapy session to talk about my experiences and what I have been through. There have been times in my life—as a child, as a young adult, and now as an adult—that I have thought I would feel better holding in all my emotions, holding in all my experiences, because, quite frankly, I didn't feel like anyone cared or would understand. The reality is, people do care, people do understand, and there are people with whom my words will resonate. Life experiences are still happening to me daily, and while I am better equipped to handle the chaos and all the unknowns, I will know for the rest of my life that I am much stronger for having experienced such events. My hope for you is that after reading about all the ways I discovered my inner strengths and learned to balance my weight of worth, you will look back on your life experiences and see all the ways in which you, my friend, are strong too.

Sincerely yours,
Victoria McCune

TABLE OF CONTENTS

Ch. 1 Before she knew 1

Ch. 2 She is *Strong* in her studies 13

Ch. 3 She is *Strong* for her mother 25

Ch. 4 She is *Strong* in her faith 43

Ch. 5 She is *Strong* for others 55

Ch. 6 She is *Strong* in her health 67

Ch. 7 She is *Strong* for her friends 79

Ch. 8 She is *Strong* for herself 91

Ch. 9 She is *Strong* but not finished 113

About the Author 117

CHAPTER 1
Before she knew . . .

I am not entirely sure what my birth story is, and quite frankly, I'm not sure I want to know the truth. I have asked my mom, Athena, a few times, as well as other relatives who were around when my mom found out she was pregnant. In asking, I have received several versions of my birth story. What I do know is my mom was seventeen. My mom, who had lived through more than enough trauma in her childhood, found out she would be seventeen and pregnant. She told me stories about the physicians who insisted she terminate her pregnancy because the baby she was carrying would be deformed or disabled. But my mom had already made up her mind, and no matter what I came into this world looking like, she would love me unconditionally.

My mom and my biological father, Gerald, did not stay together, and I was in elementary school when he passed away. When I was a child, Gerald and I lived in different states; I hadn't known any better to ask about him and why he was not in my life consistently. I did know he existed, however; he lived in Texas, and we still had lots of family living in Texas, with whom we kept in touch. We went to Texas every summer to visit family, and my mom made sure I saw Gerald and his family every time. We would go to dinner, exchange photos, and catch up on how I was doing in school, dance, and sports. But once we came back home to Colorado, I never felt the need to ask many questions about him. Growing up and asking about my heritage and where I came from, I found it fascinating to learn that Gerald was Native American, and his father (my grandfather) lived on an Indian reservation and was a chief, which made me—can you guess? An Indian princess. I didn't take the title too seriously as a kid, but every now and again, it was fun to remind the kids at my school that I was special because I was an Indian princess.

When I was a baby, my mom struggled to find stable housing; we had moved from Texas to Florida and then to Colorado, all by the time I was five years old. My mom, who had big dreams, cared for my younger brother, Mark, and I while also attending school herself and working multiple jobs to provide for herself and us kids. My mom was beautiful, independent, fun to be around, and a social butterfly. We kids were her pride and joy, and she made sure we would be safe and that we had what we needed to succeed in life. As far back as I can remember, I called my mom strong because I could sense something was never quite right with her. As a child, I knew that my mom fought demons in her mind, and while it was not always noticeable, my mom was good at putting those demons in check and carrying on with our lives. My mom, in her own skin, was strong—strong in her studies, strong as a leader, strong in her career, and strong as a single mother.

The kindergarten I attended during the week was held at the church we went to every Sunday. I watched as my mom always helped out by teaching Sunday school and youth group. As we got into middle school, she would set up retreats for our youth group to do fun activities. As we got older, helping out with our church was something I also enjoyed doing. Church was always a part of our lives growing up, and my mom continually took my brother and I, even if she didn't always have my father's support.

It wasn't until we moved to Colorado that my mom met Paul, the man my brother and I would forever call Dad. He loved us like

Ch. 1 Before she knew...

we were his own blood; his entire family accepted all of us and the way we functioned as a family. My dad would show my brother and I the importance of hard work and what it took to run a successful pizza business.

My dad, in his younger days, gushed about his sweet car—his 1990 Geo Storm. When we got to ride in his car, it was always with windows down and music up loud. But even though my dad was a guy full of fun, he and my grandfather, George, were business partners. From 1986 to 2005, they ran a pizzeria out of the Westminster Mall in Denver, Colorado. I loved being the mall rat child! I loved being able to wake up early and get to the mall before it opened, running around the food court like I owned the place. I loved the smell of my dad making the first pizza pie of the morning, which I would get to eat for breakfast. I was a short kid, and running the cash register was something I absolutely loved to do, but for me to even reach the keys, I would stand on a red plastic crate as I rang up orders for customers. I spent a lot of my weekends, summers, and holidays at the mall. On Halloween, we would dress up in our costumes and go from store to store, filling up our candy buckets. I was fascinated with learning all there was to know about making dough and pizza sauce in large quantities. Oven safety was also a part of my training early on, as we were not to be in the front of the store, jacking around by a hot oven.

Finally, in my teenage years, I was able to make pizza pies with the big boys. Not many girls liked getting dirty in flour and smelling like pizza all day, so not many girls applied for open positions. There were many days where the only people I was surrounded by were teen boys and older men who also worked for my father. Let's just say I was more than protected if my feelings ever got hurt. The days at the pizzeria were some of the best days of my life; in all honesty, it actually hurts my heart to remember those times as I write about them here in this book. As a child, I had no idea that good things don't last forever, nor did I understand that life as I knew it would be broken down into seasons.

My dad was always the "cool guy." Everyone loved him and knew him at the mall where the family business was. I, his only adopted daughter, loved my dad and was so proud to be called his daughter. Our home life was great, for the most part. I can remember our little three-bedroom house on Jackson Court. It's so true that you tend to appreciate things more when you no longer have them, and this house was no exception. Both my mom and my dad worked hard so us kids could have everything our little hearts desired. My brother started playing competitive hockey at a very young age. I myself was on a competitive dance team. Both of our activities, I realize now, were not cheap to pay for every month. But my parents never made a fuss when it came to our activities and how much they were.

The sky's the limit...

When I was a child, my family traveled a lot with my brother's hockey teams and my competitive dance studio. We would go to Cancun, Mexico, every summer, as well as Texas, Canada, California, Las Vegas in December, various cruises, and so many other places. My parents taught me that no matter how hard you work for an everyday paycheck, it is okay to work just as hard for vacations. It wasn't always easy for my dad to travel with us, because when he was gone, it was difficult to find backup to run the pizzeria. But he managed, and we made some of the best memories on those family trips. My parents were so fancy when they needed to be. Being a little girl and watching my parents get ready for dinner dates, a night out of dancing, or fancy gatherings was one of my most favorite things to do. My mom, being the lady she was, putting her makeup on just right, doing her hair, and adding her favorite perfume (Beautiful by Estee Lauder) before she left the house. Then my dad, getting on his nice dress pants and a collared shirt, then adding whatever cologne was in the bathroom at the time. I used to appreciate when my parents went on dates, because

Ch. 1 Before she knew...

that meant my brother and I would get a cool babysitter. We could stay up late, watch *South Park*, and eat my parents out of house and home.

Growing up, our home always had kids in it. We lived in a neighborhood that was blocked off from any major traffic—picture a key-shaped block. Almost every house on my childhood block had one to two kids living in the home. At one point in time, I counted over thirty kids just on our one block, which consisted of twenty-one houses; it was a busy little block, but oh, so much fun! All my friends always wanted to hang out at my house. On the Fourth of July, the adults would block off the end of our street so no one could drive in and out while we kids played and rode our bikes. At nighttime, all the families would come out front to watch the dads and teen boys light off fireworks. On Easter, my mom and her two best friends would throw an Easter brunch, and we would have ladies in the kitchen cooking egg bakes and quiches and cutting fresh fruit—all sorts of people would come into our home and dine in our tiny kitchen just to have a meal with us. Christmas was no different and was always my mom's favorite holiday. She would have decorations galore; our Christmas tree was always full and complete with a matching tree skirt. The smell of Pine-Sol, vanilla, and cinnamon lingered in our house. My mom would have a tree-trimming party every year. She would buy special ornaments for all of our friends and family and wrap them up nicely just to have everybody unwrap their ornaments and hang them on our tree. Afterwards, we kids would retreat with our friends to our rooms or to the basement and let the adults have their time.

Although I can vividly remember all the good times we had, we often had our seasons of bad times as well. My mom suffered from severe migraines that would often lay her up in bed for days at a time. I can remember being in elementary school, and some days after school, I would have to sit in the office with my younger brother while someone would call my mom to come pick us up. My mom tried so hard to be there for everything, but when she was sick, boy was she sick. As a seven-year-old kid, I was very wise and knowledgeable when it came to calling 911 and having my script ready for them when my mom would drop down to the floor and start shaking uncontrollably. Once the ambulance came and got my mom, I was the one who would call my dad and tell him where my mom was going; then I would get myself and my brother over to the neighbor's house until my parents were able to figure out a babysitting arrangement. As a young child, I never panicked while handling emergencies that involved my mom. I just made sure that when issues came up, I was helpful, I kept myself and my brother safe, and I tried to be the least of my parents' worries in the moment. I never heard my dad complain or say hurtful words; he dealt the best way he knew how, living with a woman who was, to some extent, disabled. My dad showed me strength in all the ways he silently showed up.

The struggle is real...

Teenage years, hormones, rebellion—you name it, and I'm sure I lived it. I would quickly learn all about boys, relationships, how to drive, and figuring out who I was as a person. While I had a lot of wild experiences in my teenage years, there were areas I was sure to stay away from, such as drugs. But Cupid figured out my weakness, and I experienced my first heartbreak my freshman year of high school, and then again my sophomore year with the same boy. Every boy who came after my first real boyfriend was the rebel type.

I can recall my mom needing to go in for surgery and my mother's mom—whose name is Margaret, but we call her Mema—flying into Colorado to care for my brother and I; leave it to me to sneak a boy through my front door and have him stay the night in my bed. I obviously didn't think that one through as to how I would get the boy out the next morning, since Mema would be at our house

Ch. 1 Before she knew...

all day. Needless to say, I got caught and was grounded for what I thought was a lifetime.

My teenage years brought so many changes to our family. My brother, whose life was taken over by hockey, was sent to state after state for an entire school year at a time to billet with other families so he could play hockey. I quit dance in my teenage years to start cheerleading and playing tennis more seriously. I was determined to get college scholarships playing tennis.

In these years, the family business at the pizzeria was still going strong, but the signs of changing times were slowly growing evident, and my dad had to take on a second job at the airport to offset the money that was no longer coming into our household. My mom's health during these years was also declining, showing more and more that something was just not right, and her old methods of keeping her demons in check were no longer working like they once had. We learned why my mom would have drop-down, shaking convulsions, also known as seizures. She'd tried all kinds of medications to get those under control. The migraines that once kept her laid up for days at a time were caused by a pituitary tumor. Botox treatments were used to ease those debilitating symptoms. But still, something was not right—her mind was not sharp like it had once been, and it was now starting to affect how she worked, her relationships with her friends, and her relationship with my dad.

As a teenager, my life moved forward. I was already a very independent child, and that independence took off once I received my driver's license. I was now able to get myself to and from school and practice. My brother ended up moving back to Colorado, and it was my job to get us back and forth to school and, many times, to get my brother back and forth to hockey practices or games. But I didn't mind helping my parents, because I was given all sorts of opportunities to drive my red 1998 Volkswagen Beetle. I still love that car.

My junior year of high school would prove to be the end of my childhood stability and the start of new beginnings; my parents finally chose to sell our little house on Jackson Court. I was devastated with this news, and being my teenage self, I told them both how terrible of a decision this was. I'd grown up in that house, my friends and I had written all sorts of things in my bedroom closet (graffiti, really), and the years' worth of memories extended to the rest of the house too. People knew how to find us if they needed us because we'd lived at that house so long. But my mom now needed more help at home; she was deteriorating quickly, and I couldn't begin to understand why. This was the first time I remember hearing the *c* word (cancer). My mom, come to find out, had been struggling with breast cancer and undergoing treatment and doctors' appointments all alone. I'm not sure if she ever told my dad, and he just didn't know how to respond, but I myself had not been informed, or I would have responded to the news of moving differently. At least, I hope I would have.

My mother showed me strength in fighting the cancer alone for about a year before any of us really knew what was going on. My parents sold our house on Jackson Court, and we moved to a new and bigger house in Thornton, Colorado. Our great-aunt Jill moved in with us, as my mom and her were best friends at the time. This new house would provide all of us with new beginnings, something we all longed for so badly.

The tides of change...

Around the time we moved into the new house, my brother started experiencing an identity crisis. He was asking a lot of questions about his biological dad and where he came from. The man we'd called Dad for all these years was indeed our stepdad who had legally adopted us, but my brother was adamant to figure out his own missing puzzle piece. My mom made some phone calls, and while she was still undergoing chemo treatments and losing her

Ch. 1 Before she knew...

hair, she and my brother headed off to Florida to meet my brother's biological father.

At this point in my life, I realized why I struggled with love and relationships. Although I had grown up with married parents for a majority of my life, I had never sat down to think about my mom and her past relationships. Why did my brother and I have different dads? When did that all happen? I must have met my brother's dad at some point, because I was the older sibling. What the heck was happening? Why did my mom agree to go find my brother's biological dad? I had so many questions and no one to ask. But I was a teenager, with a teenager's brain, who didn't sit and ponder something for too long before it became an afterthought.

I can't tell you exactly when my mom and brother got back from Florida or when my mom and dad had "the talk" and decided to split up, but it happened. My mom reconnected with my brother's biological father, and he planned to move from Florida to Colorado to see where his relationship with my mom would go, as well as his relationship with us kids. I coped with the situation the best way I knew how—by staying in relationships with toxic people. I coped, knowing I would soon be graduating high school, and I would no longer be in that household, dealing with the chaos. In the end, that's exactly what I was doing—just coping. My mom was soon placed in remission from her breast cancer. She underwent a double mastectomy and reconstructive surgery. The cancer had caused her to lose weight and lose her hair, but the remission brought back my spunky little mother, and her strength was evident even in her cool, spiky little hairdos.

Can you believe it...?

Although I was never into experimenting with drugs, I knew they existed, and during my mom's cancer battle, I learned why access to medical marijuana could be beneficial. While battling cancer, my mom experienced a lot of pain and nausea; smoking marijuana was her only escape. We kids did not grow up around drugs, so watching my mom smoke weed and act so strangely afterwards was awkward for me. Then add watching her do that with some of my close friends, and I became mad and irritated. My brother and I always had the "cool parents," but knowing my mom was smoking weed with some of my best friends was not at all "cool" in my eyes. But the more I saw how it helped my mom escape the pain, the less I made such a big deal out of it, not only with my mom but with my friends.

High school graduation was an amazing day; the weather was nice, and my brother's biological dad had bought me my graduation dress, which was from my favorite store, Express. It had a cute pink-and-white polka-dot belt. The dress went to my knees, and I had cute wedges to wear with it. The day was filled with lots of excitement, and we had so much family in town from all over the States. It was graduation day! I could not care less what love triangle was going on at the time; all I knew was this was the moment I had been waiting for. My freedom would be here before I knew what to do with it. I had been accepted to the University of Colorado Boulder with many scholarships to pay for my stay, and I would be moving onto the college campus in August, after the summer break. I was so happy! Walking up to get my high school diploma, I knew right then and there I wanted to experience this feeling again. My parents threw an awesome graduation party and allowed me to go to Puerto Vallarta for my senior trip. Since I clung to toxic relationships at that time, my boyfriend would also be going with me on my senior trip.

Teenage girls and their boyfriends on senior trips—I can't say it's something I will allow my own son to experience when he is older, as peer pressure and temptations happen the moment you get off the airplane. The entire group was given the rules for how the trip would go. We were given all the reasons why buying beer was a bad idea and were told that taking it back to our hotel rooms was

Ch. 1 Before she knew...

not allowed. Most of us were eighteen, and peer pressure sucked. It wasn't long before my group of friends and our boyfriends had the bright idea to do exactly what we were told not to do. We knew we wouldn't be able to smuggle beer into the hotel through the front door, so we devised a plan. Our boyfriends agreed to buy the beer off of hotel property, and we girls were instructed to wait outside, within the fences of the hotel property. The guys would meet us at the fence, fill our backpacks with the beer, and pass the backpacks to us through the fence. Then we could head to our hotel rooms and drink. All went according to plan until the very last moment. We got the beer in our backpacks and through the gated fence, but when the guys left to enter the hotel through the front door, us girls were stopped by security and asked to hand over our backpacks. Scared to death, we did as we were told. No questions asked. The guys then showed up after security, wondering where the bags were. We told them what happened.

"Yes, we gave them our bags."

"Well, did you at least grab your passports, your money, or any identifying information so you can get back home?"

"Well, no, we forgot that part."

I'm not sure how long our group searched for those security men, but thankfully, the guys found our bags in some trash bags, and we were able to continue on with our senior trip. We were never given an explanation for how we'd been caught, but we just assumed that our efforts to circumvent the rules had been caught on camera.

The summer before my freshman year of college flew by and showed me freedom in all areas of my life. I spent a lot of my time at the mall, as our days were numbered before my grandfather and my dad would have to close down the pizzeria forever. I will never forget the last day I spent in the back of that store. I had never seen the back room look so empty before. I had never felt the ovens so cold. The space where our family business had sat for nineteen years would close forever and would take all my childhood memories with it. In that moment, I learned what it meant to be strong throughout change.

CHAPTER 2
She is *Strong* in her studies . . .

As a child, I always loved school. In elementary school, I was the one who went over the top on all my projects and begged my teacher to assign me some helpful tasks to do around my classroom. School was always something that intrigued me, and although not all subjects came to me quickly, I studied and studied until I made the grades I wanted. My parents always wanted what was best for my brother and I. Going to college after high school was a given for both of us, and honestly, I enjoyed school so much I took for granted that college was what all kids did after high school. I remember attending a summer Upward Bound program at the University of Colorado Boulder. I was able to spend six weeks experiencing college life. We lived in the dorms, ate in the dining halls, and attended classes in real college classrooms; the classes we got to participate in were also transferrable as college credits.

I had always enjoyed writing and excelled in my English classes all through grade school, and CU Boulder had an amazing reputation for their journalism program. Let's just say, students were taken very seriously in the real world if they graduated from CU's journalism program, and I wanted that journalism degree more than anything. By the time I graduated high school and entered college, I had already earned enough college credits to jump into the journalism study program as a sophomore. I was thrilled. Since I was going to a major university, and that was not going to be cheap at all, my mom helped me write scholarship letters to businesses, churches, and bars, because any scholarship amount, big or small, could help pay for my tuition. It was a good idea, and those scholarships did help me pay, but I would quickly learn about financial aid and what it meant to accumulate student loan debt.

Can you stay focused...?

My freshman year of college, I was set to move into the dorms at CU Boulder and live with three other female roommates. Two of my roommates were girls I'd gone to high school with, and I was really glad to not be sharing this experience with complete strangers. I remember the day I moved into my dorm—emotions were running high as my mom went crazy and bought me everything she thought a freshman girl would need to survive without her parents: new bedding, a shower caddy complete with all the essentials, and mace. Our dorm had its own kitchen and bathroom; it really was our very own apartment. We needed dishes, glassware, silverware, groceries, and so much stuff just to make this place livable. Then came orientation, where we received our class schedules for the semester.

After attending my first college class in an auditorium that held more than three hundred students, I realized that the professors rarely knew their students by name, and they couldn't care less if we came to class or not. There was no hand-holding in how they rolled out the syllabi, showing us detailed breakdowns of what the semester would hold. Sitting in my first astronomy class, I received the syllabus and realized that chapters one and two were supposed

Ch. 2 She is *Strong* in her studies...

to be read by the first day of class. All I could think was, "Shit, I'm already behind." I hadn't even bought textbooks yet. Needless to say, coming from a relatively small high school with a graduating class of 120, I was not at all prepared to attend such a big university. Even the Upward Bound program could not have prepared me for the amount of traffic I would experience on campus every day.

Days came and went, and soon I realized the true expense of being a college student; I needed to get a job. I did what everyone else my age was doing and went to the closest mall, found one of my favorite stores, and applied for a job. I'd had previous work experience at our family restaurant, so that helped my application, and before I knew it, I was hired and making $5.50 an hour. My new employer was great about working with my school schedule, and I felt fearless because here I was, living the dream, or so I thought.

During this time, my parents were fully immersed in their divorce, and my brother had moved again to another state and was billeting with a family while he played competitive hockey. I endured my first semester of college as well as a working freshman could, but money was tight, and I had stuff I needed to buy. I was so torn on whom to ask for money, as my parents' divorce seemed to be weighing on both my mom and my dad. That's when I took on cleaning houses. At first I started doing it just for friends who needed me here and there, but then word got out that this was my new gig, and before long, I had quite a few clients who would pay me to clean their houses.

My next semester in college proved to be harder than the first semester; you can imagine why, with me working two jobs and still trying to keep up with fifteen credit hours in school. Needless to say, I ended the semester with a few Fs. I had never failed a class before, and it wasn't like high school, where the teachers call your parents to report you for not turning in homework or for doing poorly on a test—no, not like that at all. Instead, I alone would know I'd received an F. I could hold the news all to myself, and no one would have to know. That was, until I was placed on academic probation and would also have to report the failed grades to the businesses that had given me scholarships.

It was humiliating for me to admit I'd failed at the one task I'd been sent to do, which was to go to school and earn good grades. I'm sure I could have been a bit more rational and not have taken the failing grades so hard—heck, our family was going through some major life changes, and I would have had every right to blame my problems on my parents' rocky relationship, but I didn't do that. Instead, I would have to repeat classes, and graduation was no longer looking attainable in the next four years. I took the failing grades rather hard. But it was about to be summertime, and my two jobs were still going strong; at least I was excelling in one area of my life.

After my first year living in the dorms and leaving for summer break, my mother and I decided it would be best financially—and maybe not so distracting for me—if I commuted to college for my second year at CU Boulder. My mom could also use my help at home, since her health, while not terrible, was not great, as she struggled with depression and anxiety. Plus, I was in a new relationship, and living in the dorms would keep my new boyfriend and I apart more than we wanted. I kept the job at the mall, but I did let my job cleaning houses go for good to prevent me from getting behind in my studies again. My second year attending CU Boulder did not seem to be any easier for me; for once in my life, school was really hard for me. Nothing I could do would help me earn the grades I was used to making. I'd graduated high school with honors, and now that I was in college, I felt dumb and very much uneducated and out of place. I still held on to the dream of being a traveling journalist for *National Geographic*, but no one was going to hire a girl who couldn't pass her media classes.

It was around this time that I applied for an internship with KUSA, a local television company. My grades were definitely not appealing to them, but maybe my story would be, or so I thought. It would be an internship, unpaid for two semesters (not that I could afford that), but it would give me experience in a local newsroom. I was all about utilizing experiences so I could add them to my resume. This internship was highly discussed among most of the journalism majors, and while most kids who attended CU Boulder did not have all the personal issues I was dealing with, a lot of them got accepted for this internship. I had to sit on the sidelines, watching everyone else make their dreams come true.

I realized how truly unfair life can be. No one cared or asked me about my dreams; instead, I would have to put all my dreams on hold and reevaluate. Plus, my mom's mental health was declining, and she had become much more forgetful. My relationship with my dad was now put on the back burner because I was so hurt he'd left our family and was rarely keeping in touch with me. He'd left me, and now my brother's billet family was calling my phone because their monthly billet fee was no longer getting paid. In so many areas of my life, we were failing as a family—all at once. I ended my second year of college with more Fs, and no one cared. No one asked me about it, so I never talked about it.

One step forward, ten steps back...

The only thing going right at this point was the relationship I was in with a boy named Alex. He listened to me, he kept me focused on our future together, and he would truly make me forget about all my worries. We talked about our future a lot and decided it was best if we just moved in together. He was older than me, and he had a credit score (this was a big deal). My mom was okay with this plan as long as the two of us bought something—no renting. So off we went, house hunting, until we found a cute two-bedroom condo close to my mom's house, and we were able to get approved for a $150,000 mortgage loan! It was, at the time, a steal of a deal. We were so excited!

I would need to find a higher-paying job, because now we had a mortgage, so I quit my job at the mall and found a banking position close to our new condo. I got so wrapped up in my new life with my boyfriend that when school was set to start back up again, I was not enrolled anywhere. I had not taken the steps I needed to get off academic probation. Heck, I think that buried deep in my school emails was an announcement from admissions stating that they'd actually kicked me out of college. But I didn't care; my new life and new focus were looking better than anything a college degree could give me.

My boyfriend would soon turn into my husband, and we'd go shopping every weekend—no exaggeration. He would take me dancing, and we would go to fancy dinners. He was great with money, or so I thought, since he had amazing credit. He always had new cars, complete with upscale rims, tires, and, of course, a sound system. He was so cool. I loved our life we were making together.

We would live our lives this way for a few years. It's okay to call me naive now, but I certainly didn't realize it then, and eventually all that spending would catch up with us. I remember the day we sat down to go over our finances, and he suggested we rent out our condo for a while so we could focus on paying off some debt.

"Wait, what do you mean, debt?" I asked him. We both worked full time, my checks were direct deposit, and he handled all the bills. I didn't handle this talk with him very well. I was even more furious at him since he had already done the legwork to have our condo rented out, and now we needed to agree on moving back in with his parents. Like an ashamed dog, I stuck my tail between my legs and asked my mom and Aunt Jill if I could move back in with them. My mom—of course, being my biggest cheerleader—agreed, but my great-aunt was not having my news. She was accustomed to a controlled, restricted home life, and my unexpected news threatened to disrupt their stability and add an unpredictable factor to the mix. This led to a huge family fight. Ultimately, my mom had

Ch. 2 She is *Strong* in her studies...

to choose her daughter over my great-aunt and her rules, which meant my mom, her boyfriend, and I had to find a new place to live, and quickly. We found a cute house in Commerce City, Colorado, where we could finally all live freely. During this time, I tried to pick up the pieces of my broken heart and reevaluate my goals. My husband and I separated and ultimately ended up going through the divorce process that caused us to file for bankruptcy. Great! Now, at twenty-two years old, I had been married, divorced, bankrupt, and a college dropout. What a track record. The only stability I felt I could cling to was my job, and oh, did I love my banking job.

Remember when I said college would be the start of me learning about student loans? Turns out, loans need to be paid back, and the government does indeed expect you to pay them back, even if you have nothing to show for them. I had to make a decision, and that involved me facing my fear of being a college dropout. I figured that if I was going to do college and not fail, I would need to go about it slower than I had the first time. Going back to CU Boulder was not an option for me, so I enrolled at my local college, Metro State University, in downtown Denver. Turns out, when you fail at one university, no matter how many years have gone by, your past catches up with you. To apply for the new school, I had to write multiple letters explaining to admissions why they should accept me. It was so embarrassing trying to start new and having my past come up like that. After multiple letters of recommendations and with a strict academic plan in place, I was approved to start attending Metro State.

While I still had a heart for journalism, I also knew that at some point in my life, I wanted to become a mother, and the idea of being a traveling journalist and a mother just didn't sound appealing. So, I started at Metro State by changing my major and getting into courses that would earn me my teaching degree. This time around, I focused on improving the balance between my work life and school life. I made sure I was prepared for each and every class. Class sizes were smaller at my new school, which helped me feel more welcome and not just like another number on a professor's roster. I was finally getting my groove back with making good grades. I even allowed myself to open back up to love again.

Just have patience . . .

The day I met Shawn was a day I will never forget. My girlfriend and I were all giddy about our recent skydiving experience, and we were headed to a local bar to chat it up. Shawn and his cousin were clearly at the bar to decompress after a hard day of work, as they were still in their dirty work clothes. For my girlfriend and I to sit together, we needed Shawn to move down a seat. He agreed. We got to talking—or, as I'm sure of now, I did all the talking about the crazy life I was living, how I needed to move my parents and myself that weekend, and how we had no help. Looking back, I was a complete disaster. But Shawn just listened, and then he agreed to help me move. I was ecstatic! My girlfriend, however, was convinced only a creep would be so interested in my story over a few beers, and only a creep would agree to help us move.

Either way, he showed up, and he helped us move. My friendship with Shawn quickly led to us being more than friends. He learned just how busy I truly was with work, school, my family, and my dealings with my ex-husband. There was even a time I tried to warn Shawn, telling him I was toxic, complicated, and not worth the fight. Shawn showed me strength in continuing to show up for me, day after day. He knew about my past, and that didn't bother him. Shawn made it clear in more ways than one that he was my missing puzzle piece. He supported and encouraged me with my goal to complete college.

Shawn and I shared our hopes and dreams, and while he'd rented a house with his brother for the last ten years, Shawn was ready to buy his first home. One we could share together, and I could finally

Ch. 2 She is *Strong* in her studies...

stop moving. We moved into our new home in Brighton, Colorado. It was a fixer-upper two-story home. We were happy!

Life was going as it should. I was still taking classes at Metro and making small strides that would get me to graduation—then the inevitable happened. My employer at the bank—the job I'd invested so much time and energy into, and the only stable thing in my life for the last five years—fired me. I felt as I had when I'd received an F in school, but getting fired felt even worse. I had never been fired from anything in my life before. I was, or thought I was, a great employee. I was devastated by the news, and life as I knew it stopped. I would again stop chasing my dream of a college education, because what did it matter? I was good at taking one step forward and ten steps backward. I could not afford to complete the student teaching courses without a job.

Unemployment lasted six weeks. Everyone would tell me to just enjoy my time off work, saying it was God's way of slowing me down. Honestly, even though Shawn and I pushed through as a couple during this time, enjoying unemployment was not something I mastered. I applied for anything and everything just to get myself back to work. Through it all, Shawn never bad-mouthed me; he instead listened when I needed him to and was a shoulder to cry on when I needed him most. I ended up getting hired at my local county office, helping individuals and families apply for government assistance. This was a field I had absolutely no experience in. No one in my immediate family had ever been on government assistance, as far as I knew. But hey, they hired me, and I needed a job badly, so I took it.

I worked at my local county office for six months before finding out I was pregnant. Shawn's family was somewhat old fashioned, believing that couples who had babies together should be married first. I was so nervous to tell his parents the news, especially since we had no intentions yet of getting married. We told everyone our news with the help of personalized M&M's; it worked out perfectly, but now that I was having a baby, school would be put on the back burner even longer. Our son, Urijah, was born March 1, 2013. He was perfect! Five pounds, eleven ounces. He was our baby boy, and we loved him so very much! The space that Shawn and I had shared would now be shared with our son, and boy, did that take us for a ride.

I am a dreamer...

By the time my son turned one, I still felt the longing desire, the tug at my heart, to finish college. I was convinced my college dream would never come true. How would I manage taking a full-time school schedule, being a mom, working full time, and managing our household? It was a complete overload, but I figured the only way I would succeed would be to truly take it one class at a time, so I did all the research necessary to figure out which college would accept me, especially for a degree program that would use most of the college credits I had already earned.

By the time I found Ashford University's online college program, I had been in college on and off for nine years, and in that time, I'd changed my major twice. Even though I was currently working in the human services field, I had been really good at my banking job and had discovered a passion for educating people about loans and finances. Ashford University had a business administration program with an emphasis on finance that would allow me to graduate within a reasonable amount of time and not waste credits I had already earned from the two previous colleges I had attended. The university was an accredited college based out of California and would allow me to take one class at a time. Ashford was my answer.

The counselors at that school held my hand for four years. Whenever I started feeling discouraged, they would stay on the phone with me for as long as I needed to talk myself out of quitting

Ch. 2 She is *Strong* in her studies...

school. When financial aid ran out, and I became a cash-paying student, the financial aid counselors walked me through how being a cash-paying student was doable with everything else I was facing. Time spent at the university showed me that no two professors are the same, and the professors who worked for Ashford understood the effort it took to keep students engaged in an online learning environment, which I would argue is harder than in a traditional learning environment. Every class encouraged me and pushed me to want to earn the best grades, even if that meant doing school late at night, early in the mornings, or on my laptop in a hospital room. Every step of the way, Ashford was good at keeping the bigger picture in my sights and maintaining my excitement about graduation.

October 2017—I was able to graduate from college in beautiful San Diego, California, and having my family there to support me was icing on the cake. It gave validation to the importance of following those intense tugs at my heart, confirming that I shouldn't give up on myself just because something was hard. I will never be able to thank the school enough for all the hand-holding and emotional support they gave me so I could call myself a college graduate. I truly learned what it meant to remain strong in my studies and, even with all odds against me, to be able to finish. Being strong in my studies was not easy, and it took me thirteen years to truly make that dream for myself come true. Through such a journey, I learned no one will ever care about my dreams to the extent I do, and I can't expect other people to make my dreams happen for me.

The journalism degree did not come to fruition then, but look at me now, falling back on my passion. No, I am not writing for *National Geographic* just yet, or the news, for that matter, but I do write a personal blog called *This is Me Doing Life*, and the content that I write has been viewed all over the world. That in itself is exciting and rewarding. It is not a job that pays the bills, but it is my outlet and keeps me sane most days.

Being strong in my studies then meant I never gave up when life got hard, even if that meant taking one class at a time or staying up late to make sure I turned in assignments on time. Being strong in my studies showed me that I can achieve anything I set my heart and mind to. Being strong in my studies now is helping me become a better, more educated member of society. Being strong and confident in my studies now is helping me grow in all areas of my life and learn the importance of passing knowledge down to younger generations.

CHAPTER 3
She is *Strong* for her mother...

My mom struggled with disabilities all throughout my childhood and into my adult life. She is a DES Daughter, which means she was exposed to the hormone diethylstilbestrol prior to birth—a term that is definitely worth a Google search. She has had multiple cancers due to being a DES Daughter, including stomach cancer, ovarian cancer, breast cancer, and colon cancer, just to name a few. She is without a doubt one of the strongest women I know. There comes a time, though, when even the most strong-minded people break down; their mindsets erode, and their physical bodies deteriorate and finally give way.

My mother became permanently disabled in 2006 at the age of thirty-eight; she would have to rely on a monthly social security check to provide for herself. My mom lost her ability to drive and was forced to quit her successful career as a paralegal. My mom would have to learn all her new limitations overnight, or so it felt. The adjustments were hard not only for her but for everyone else to adjust to.

No longer would my mom be able to say, "I am going to run to the store real quick." My mom would now have to communicate her every move to someone else and deal with a new stress of finding a ride for every little thing she wanted to do. This limitation alone proved to be frustrating for all of us. Money was even a subject of concern; ever since she and my dad had divorced, money had been tight for our family. Even though I was working and relatively on my own, my mom still had expenses to cover for herself.

A few years down the road, debt had accrued quickly, and it wasn't long till our rent payment was due, but there was no money in the bank for my mom to pay it. Meanwhile, I was going through my own financial issues and marital problems with Alex. My mom and I agreed it was time to help each other out and work together. We already lived together in a rental property, but I took control of all the funds coming in and the expenses going out for groceries and bills. My mom, her boyfriend, and I were able to create a budget and take control of all our outstanding debt.

Accepting the uncertainty...

It's funny to reflect on how life works out, especially in seasons of doubt. Our family was in a season where year after year, we lived a life of craziness, but it was clear our family bond was strong; it was clear we all needed one another to get through such hard times. I was blessed to be able to live with my mom and her boyfriend, Jimmy (whom I now call my stepdad), and truly get to know who he was as a person. My stepdad is my brother's biological father. He also has a daughter, Karen, who is in between my brother and I in age. She herself was not so fortunate in her childhood and was sucked into a life of drugs and prostitution. Leave it to good ole social media to bring to light that my stepdad's daughter was alive, sober, and in prison for various crimes and drug charges. She was scheduled to be released in late 2010 but had no family to whom she could be released.

Ch. 3 She is *Strong* for her mother...

We were given my stepsister's address in jail so we could write letters back and forth to see if our family could help her once she was released from prison. My family was not entirely open to the idea of writing to this girl, due to her history, so I took it upon myself to write the first letter. In our letters, back and forth, I learned my stepsister was a drug addict; she'd had five babies and had lost custody of all of them due to her addiction and her subsequent actions. This prison sentence was the longest she had served. She was determined to stay clean once released, but she would need to get out of Texas to ensure she would not fall back into bad habits. My mom and stepdad agreed to allow her to stay with them in their home, which I no longer lived in, once she was released. The arrangement worked for a few months, but it was not enough to keep my stepsister clean and away from temptation. She found all the bad people in our local city; she spiraled down quickly and ended up running back to Texas to her old stomping grounds.

In 2011, my niece, Hope Grace, was born in the state of Texas. She was such a beautiful baby. My mom and stepdad were notified of the new baby and were asked, since my stepdad was legally her grandfather, if they would be willing to take her.

"Of course," my mom immediately replied. My mom had always felt her best contribution to the world was raising kids. I, however, was not so sure any of this was a good idea, but I was also not in a position where I myself was ready to take on a new baby. I gave my mom all the reasons why she shouldn't agree to take on my niece. Did my mom not remember everything she'd put me through as a young child? Did my mom think that was okay or, better yet, normal for a young child to live with? I was grown now, but while I had been growing up, had my mom ever thought about what our childhood experiences were like? As the older sister, I'd always protected my younger brother. I'd never wanted Mark to experience the difficulties we faced as a family, either with health or money. By the time Hope Grace was born, though, I no longer lived with my mom and stepdad, and I wouldn't be able to protect my niece when something bad happened or when my mom experienced a bad health day.

My niece, Hope Grace, was born a drug baby. She would have to be detoxed for days, alone in the NICU. She was in Texas, and we lived in Colorado—talk about feeling helpless! Once detoxed, my niece would be released to a foster mom, who would take care of her until my mom and stepdad could get all the legalities completed with not only Texas Child Protective Services but also Colorado Child Protective Services. My mom and stepdad went through home visits, CBI checks, a detailed interview, and lots and lots of paperwork to prove they were fit enough to care for a baby.

In early February, after a very detailed review of our entire lives, Hope Grace was flown to Colorado with a social worker and given a new home with our family. While I have always been in her life since day one, I still wasn't entirely convinced this was the best decision, but a judge reviewed her case, and it was clear we'd passed all evaluations and home visits for my niece to be here. I had experience with babies, as I have lots of younger cousins, but with those babies, you could send them home after you'd given them all kinds of candy. Hope Grace, fondly nicknamed Gracie, was legally my parent's responsibility, but it would truly take a village to raise her. My then boyfriend and now husband, Shawn, was so supportive of my family during this time; I loved watching him interact with my niece. We would often babysit her on the weekends to give my parents a much-needed break. We had just bought our first home together, and life was moving as it should.

As both our hearts opened for Gracie, it didn't take much discussion for Shawn and I to start thinking about starting a family of our own. Urijah Gage was born on March 1, 2013. He came into the world screaming. Our family was feeling completely full with all this baby love.

Ch. 3 She is *Strong* for her mother...

Gracie and Urijah would grow up having the best of both worlds—being able to relate to each other like brother and sister while also being able to retreat to separate homes when they were done playing with one another. Our kids would share birthday celebrations, holidays, vacations, church, and summer programs with each other, and we wouldn't have had it any other way. Raising our kids together would show me strength as I learned that the life we live every day is not at all about me. Life as we know it is not meant to be lived in isolation; it is meant to be shared in community with others. The strength I learned from my niece, Gracie, who started out her life literally fighting to live until she came out on the other side is hard to describe, along with the strength I learned from my son, who has shown me patience and love in a way I never knew possible. I will forever be grateful God called me to be Urijah's mommy and Gracie's forever friend.

Let go and let God . . .

The year 2016 would change all of our lives forever. My mom, who for years had been dealing with epilepsy, had an implant in her back that would help control bowel function. Little did we know at the time, but this device malfunctioned and almost killed her, causing her to have twenty or more seizures in one day. She had been in the hospital five days before everyone realized the seizures would subside once the device was turned off. Turned off meant no bowel control—can you imagine no bowel control or function? Not being able to feel when you have to go to the bathroom? It was awful for my mom and for our family, who had to see her basically be a guinea pig for science until her doctors could figure out what the next move would be. Finally, we saw a colon and rectal surgeon who agreed my mom would be the best candidate for a permanent ostomy. Put simply, an ostomy is a surgically created opening in the stomach, which allows for stool to pass through and be collected in an ostomy bag. The surgeon agreed this would provide my mom with a better quality of life; it was a risky surgery, but it could really change my mom's life once she adjusted to having it. I'd never thought taking a poop the traditional way was something I took for granted, but after hearing the details of the surgery and what they would have to do to create an ostomy, I quickly realized how something so simple as taking a poop in the toilet was truly a luxury.

My mom gave the idea some thought, and through the tears, she agreed this was her only solution to getting back to living. My mom would have this big operation a week before Christmas; mind you, we still had two babies at home, both with lots of questions as to why Mimi (a.k.a., my mom) was so sick and in the hospital so often lately. We still had Christmas traditions we needed to follow through with, as Christmas was my mom's favorite holiday. The day of the big surgery, I remember feeling overwhelmed and really nervous. After the nurses prepped my mom for surgery, it came time to say our goodbyes. I knew the next time I would see my mom, she would have a bag permanently attached to her tummy. During her surgery, I prayed a lot, I cried, and I questioned God and his intentions regarding this season we were in.

Why my mom? Her life was filled with so much suffering. Why make one person endure so much suffering? One Bible story I'd heard over and over again during this time of my life was the book of Job. Job was a successful man in the Bible. He had it all—wealth, family, money. Job was a man of God and trusted God deeply. God allowed Satan to test Job, but Satan was not allowed to kill him. Satan started by killing all Job's children, taking away his family, and then giving him unimaginably poor health. Job continued to claim his love for the Lord and refused to sin against the Lord. Because of Job's obedience to the Lord, God allowed Job to heal and be blessed; despite all Job had lost, God doubled Job's blessings later on in his life.

Ch. 3 She is *Strong* for her mother...

The Job Bible story was always on my mind in real time, especially when it came to my mom. My mom grew up in church, she went to a Catholic school, and she was, for the longest time, a woman of God, but she'd lost her faith somewhere along the way. In her mind, God was absent. She was angry and upset; God seemed absent in a time when she needed to feel him the most. My questions would remain unanswered during this surgery, but knowing Job could live through all of Satan's trials gave me hope for my mom and her situation. My mom came out of surgery, and what do you know, she was actually in good spirits. She learned all about her new ostomy and what her new routine would look like. She had to stay in the hospital a few days to make sure the ostomy worked how it should.

The surgery was a success, and my mom got to go home with the help of home healthcare, of course. Scheduling when the nurses would come do home visits, planning physical therapy appointments, and having my mom meet with an ostomy specialist proved a full load in itself. But as a family, we were all willing to help in any way we could. Mema came out to stay with my mom, stepdad, and my niece for a month so I could have a bit of a break each day and be able to focus on my studies. Overall, my mom was adjusting well and making great strides in learning all there was to learn about having an ostomy. How to dress it properly, how to look for leaks, what her diet needed to consist of. She was doing really well. Then came time to introduce full-body showers. My mom was terrified! This whole device would have to shower with her, and she was worried about so many things, most of all whether the experience would be painful. A home health nurse walked her through all the steps. Ostomies are tricky, as moisture anywhere near an ostomy is like a breeding ground for nasty bacteria; it only takes a few hours for a moist area to break out in a full-blown wound when you have an ostomy.

Even as my mom was making amazing strides in learning how to maneuver life with an ostomy, she developed the most painful wound around her new stoma, the man-made opening in her large intestine that allowed stool to exit her body. Witnessing her pain and constant need for lidocaine to even touch or dress the wound was hard for me. It took my mom six months of wound-care appointments to fully get this raging wound under control and closed up. The kids, at this point, used the word *ostomy* in their everyday vocabulary and could tell you why people have them and what comes out of them.

Our family tried to find humor in our chaos. We encouraged my mom to name her stoma, and because there was no control over the random noises the stoma would make, we would all giggle when her stoma decided to be vocal, always catching us by surprise. Some days were better than others, and just when we thought my mom's health was getting back on track, she would face another hurdle. My mom had not been maintaining potassium levels ever since she got her ostomy. It took five ER visits and hospital admissions to figure out my mom would need to be on a regular potassium supplement to keep her out of the hospital and stabilize her potassium levels. For months, it seemed like I was living hour by hour, because if I began to envision a full day without some sort of setback, a setback was sure to happen. We lived this way for months, taking it hour by hour and day by day with my mom.

Let the tears flow . . .

In July 2017, my mom was spending an afternoon in a canoe, fishing with my stepdad. My mom had been experiencing numbness in her left side for a few days before the incident happened. The feeling would come and go, but nothing could have prepared us for my mother's next medical emergency. The numbness coming and going was an indication my mom was experiencing a stroke, and when the full stroke hit her body, there was no stopping it. She managed to call 911 and get help. I rushed to the hospital once I

Ch. 3 She is *Strong* for her mother...

found out. When I made it to my mom, she was completely paralyzed on her left side.

The ER doctor made it clear to our family she would need to administer TPA (tissue plasminogen activator). This medication could potentially stop the clot, which could, over time, help my mom make a full recovery from the stroke; however, TPA didn't have a huge success rate for people with a history of cancer. I was my mother's legal power of attorney, and although she was conscious and could speak for herself, it was up to me to make the decision to give her such a powerful medication. If we chose not to give my mom the medication, she would probably never be able to walk again or feed herself again, and if we opted for the medication, we would risk her bleeding out due to the weak tissue in her body from receiving chemo and radiation in the past. The list of restrictions went on and on. Since my mom could still speak and understand the extent of what was going on, we all knew giving my mom the drug was necessary, and whatever happened in between, we would face it together.

Our family agreed for her to have the drug, and we would know her fate within a few hours of the medication being given to her. This was another moment for me where I thought about Job's story and questioned God's timing. Why would he continue to allow my mom to suffer?

I'm not proud I prayed this prayer, but as her last twelve months had not been a cakewalk, I began to pray, "God, please end her suffering. It's not fair to her. I will be sad to no longer have my mom, but I don't want her to suffer anymore." I prayed this partly out of selfishness, wanting so badly to be done with hospitals. I didn't want to watch my mom suffer unbearable pain; I wanted for our kids to no longer wonder what family member would be at our doorstep next to offer help because they knew Mimi was sick again.

I cried a lot during this season. God didn't answer my prayer that day; instead, he sent a miracle. My mom survived her stroke in July 2017. After a hospital stay of a few days, she was sent to an inpatient rehab center, where they helped her work on mobility on her left side. It was there she had to relearn how to walk as she restrengthened the left side of her body.

At this point, I was juggling my final semester of college, my mom's health, my full-time job, and being a mama and a wife. My mom went into the rehab center not walking on her own, and my mind raced with all the what-ifs. She lived in a two-story home with no bathroom on the main floor—what if she could never go up the stairs again? Would she need someone to be with her 24-7 once she was released?

I questioned all my daily priorities at this point. Should I keep my full-time job? Should I stay enrolled in school? Was there too much going on for the kids to handle? But my mom needed me to stay strong for her when she couldn't be strong for herself. I never prayed for help, but God knows our needs before we can say them out loud. He showed me loud and clear I was not doing this alone. I had never met anyone in my stepdad's family; I had rarely even heard him speak about them in the thirteen years he and my mom had been back together. My help would come to me and my family through my stepdad's mother. Her loved ones all called her Nanny. She was an awesome lady!

Truly, God's timing couldn't have been more perfect. She was able to stay with my mom, my stepdad, and my niece for a month and a half after my mom was released from rehab. I will always call her my angel, because she literally had nothing else to give our family other than her help, and I so needed an extra set of hands. We still had kids to get back and forth from the bus stop, meals to prep and prepare, and household chores to keep up with, as well as making sure my mom was taking her medications properly and doing her exercises. Nanny coming to help my family allowed me

Ch. 3 She is *Strong* for her mother...

to stay enrolled in school and not quit. With Nanny's help, I no longer had to devote all my time to the care of my mom. I could now handle the task of finishing up my final assignments, knowing my mom was safe and cared for with Nanny staying by her side. I learned strength from a woman I'd just met; she packed up her life to help a family in need, for no other reason than that she could. Thank you so much, Nanny!

October 2017—San Diego, here we come. I graduated college. A thirteen-year journey, and I literally had to kick, scream, and cry to make it happen. My mom was only a few months out from her stroke episode, and we were unsure if the doctor would even allow her to go on an airplane to attend my graduation ceremony. We would not find out that news until a week before we were set to fly out. We bought my mom an airline ticket just in case she got the all clear to travel, and we purchased travel insurance just in case it was not possible. To our surprise, she was cleared to go.

Confidence is beautiful...

Our family flew to San Diego, and for the first time in two years, we were not worried about my mom's health. Our kids got to be kids, I got to enjoy my husband, and I got to truly embrace the moment and give myself the grace I deserved for getting through all the crap. My heart was still beating, I'd persevered, I'd finally done it, and dang it, I was proud of myself.

Going to college had consumed a lot of my time, and my family had often sacrificed spending time with me just so I could get an assignment done and turned in on time. My husband, Shawn, who was an amazing partner to tackle such a big dream with, took on being a dad and son-in-law with such charm. I'm sure there were days and weekends when he felt lonely and overwhelmed with the kids, but he was such a trooper, never complaining when my school workload took over.

We finished 2017 strong and confident as a family after overcoming so many hurdles. We knew life wasn't perfect, but after being tested and put through the ringer and coming out the other side, I was sure our family would finally get the quality time we all deserved with one another.

For a short time, my mother's health was stable. She was adjusting to her ostomy and getting the hang of all her new medications. However, my mom continually insisted that she was feeling overmedicated most days. Getting her physicians to back off on medications was never an easy task. When I say my family was always good at taking one step forward and ten steps back, January 2018 would prove to be no different.

Persevering through pain . . .

My mom, God bless her, had every right to not like where she was in life; she had every right to be angry at the world. In January, my mom continually kept telling her physicians she was feeling overmedicated, but since she has preexisting health conditions, my mom will need certain medications for the rest of her life to keep her health problems in check.

I was at church one Sunday morning—I'd known my mom was having a hard morning, but to keep some normalcy for my son and my niece, we'd agreed to attend church. Service wasn't even ten minutes in before my phone rang. It was the Walmart pharmacy, saying my mom had called them, slurring her words, and someone needed to get to her as soon as possible. I quickly gathered my things and left my stepdad, my husband, and the kids behind at church so I could get to my mom.

The fifteen-minute drive to my mom's house felt like an eternity. What would I walk in on once I got to her house? What had she done? I was not at all prepared to see my mom in the shape she

Ch. 3 She is *Strong* for her mother...

was in. My mom was on the floor, hunched over, vomiting, with a huge, tennis ball–size bump on her left eyebrow from falling. I had seen her body shaking before, but this seemed different. I immediately called 911; they tried to keep me calm, but I was not at all calm. I just wanted them to hurry, to come help me. I kept looking at this giant bump on her eyebrow. She had fallen before, but she'd never fallen hard enough to create such a massive bump.

While I was on the phone with 911, my mom went lifeless, the throwing up stopped, and the convulsing ceased. My adrenaline was pumping. Was I even feeling her pulse, or was that the beat of my own heart? I was so scared; I felt so alone.

Finally, the ambulance and medics arrived at my mom's house, and one medic immediately began CPR and chest compressions while another medic was instructed to push on the massive bump on her head and hold on tight. I was instructed to gather up all her medications and insurance cards.

My mom was rushed to the closest hospital in Brighton because, as the medics informed me, she was coding and needed help right away. I knew it was bad when the medics would not even let me ride in the ambulance. They advised me to meet them at the hospital instead. After gathering my things and all my mom's necessities, I got in my car and rushed to the hospital, taking as many deep breaths as I could to keep myself from crying.

I arrived at the hospital and ran through the ER doors. I was stopped by a receptionist asking which patient I was there for, what her birthday was, and how she got there. Oh my goodness, why all the questions? To make matters worse, I was asked to take a seat and wait for a nurse to come out and get me.

Finally, someone came and got me. The doctor needed to speak with me. While six to seven people worked on my mom in the big ER procedure room, I was asked about my mom's medical history and the medications she was on. Since I was the one who took her to all her appointments, I knew the answers, but I was not at all ready to hear what they thought was happening to my mom.

I learned my mom was experiencing an overdose of prescription medications. The hospital we were at would do everything they could to get her stable, which involved pumping her stomach multiple times to get out all the pills, inserting an IV through a main artery in her leg, and getting her on life support to help her oxygen levels stay consistent and prevent permanent brain injury. Once she was stable, she would be transferred by helicopter to a bigger facility with an ICU unit to monitor her.

It was a lot of information to take in. The doctor did make it clear as well that if my mom passed away at any point of transport, her insurance may not cover the cost, due to this being declared as an overdose. I honestly didn't care about the cost; I just wanted my mom to be okay, and it was not clear to me at that moment that she would ever be okay again.

A transport ambulance was near the hospital and would be able to move my mom safely and on life support to a bigger Denver hospital, so the threat of a Flight for Life bill was no longer a discussion. I again could not ride with my mom and had to drive myself to the next hospital. So far, I hadn't had much time to text anyone or give updates on what was being said or done. On the car ride to the next hospital, I began to actually feel somewhat relieved to know my mom's heart was still beating, and we were going somewhere that had doctors with more experience in dealing with overdoses. My stepdad and my mom's close friend Peg would meet me in Denver so I wouldn't have to be alone.

Once my mother was admitted to the ICU, doctors asked me all the same questions: "Do you think she was trying to kill herself? Do you know what medications she is taking?"

Ch. 3 She is *Strong* for her mother...

For the rest of the night and into the next day, her care team worked closely to figure out her care plan. My mom remained in a medically induced coma to allow her brain to rest and her body to remain calm from all the trauma of the day. Family was instructed to go home and get a good night's rest. She would be cared for, and I could go back the next morning. Arriving at home that night, I was exhausted.

I remember walking out to the parking lot with my stepdad, the trooper that he was in dealing with a significant other who had disabilities, and telling him I would fully understand if he walked away and never came back. This was more than anyone could have bargained for. His words were comforting, and that night, he didn't walk away from me—that night, he told me that as a family, we would get through this together. His words will stick with me for the rest of my life. My stepdad would show me strength in staying in the chaos. He would show me strength in showing up for our family and not running away.

The next day at the hospital was emotionally draining; doctors planned to wean my mom off of life support and reverse her medically induced coma. No one was sure if she could wake up or breathe on her own, so they would have to do this process very slowly. Hour by hour, my mom was showing signs of improvement. She was waking up, still with a breathing tube in her mouth, and was terrified by all the machines. It was our job to hold her hand, whisper to her what was happening, and remind her to keep breathing and taking big breaths so she wouldn't choke or get worked up with anxiety. The process took over nine hours for her to fully wake up and keep her oxygen levels up on her own. It wasn't until late in the evening that she finally got all the heavy tubing pulled from her mouth. My mom showed me strength in listening to instructions and remaining patient during such a rigorous process.

Mema flew into town the following day, which I appreciated, knowing that once my mom was off of life support and could talk for herself, we would have to address the elephant in the room, and I wasn't convinced I wanted to address it alone. Psychiatrists streamed in and out of my mom's hospital room over the next few days to determine what had truly happened the Sunday morning my mom had almost died. Was this truly an accidental overdose, or was she really being overmedicated? As my mother's health advocate, I had been to every doctor's appointment over the past twenty-four months, and we had addressed concerns about certain medications needing to be reduced, as we'd felt the dosages were too high. But switching medications for my mom was always risky; her complications with medications proved to be life-threatening.

With the involvement of the psychiatrists, we learned that my mom had experienced a prescribed prescription overdose—a.k.a. an accidental overdose. A week before the overdose, my mom had been taken off of a seizure medication cold turkey and put on a new one that would not make her feel so loopy. The dosages were different than what she was used to—instead of a twice-a-day medication, she was supposed to take the new medication only once a day. Turned out, my mom had been trying to call the Walmart pharmacy because she'd felt funny after taking her daily medications. She knew her body well enough to know that what she was feeling was not right, but by the time she'd called the pharmacy, her airways had most likely already been closing, causing her slurred speech.

My mom was never the kind of lady to have a Monday through Sunday pillbox; she kept all her meds in a heavy-duty, reusable lime-green grocery bag. We all learned a valuable lesson from almost losing my mother that day. She was discharged from the hospital with strict guidelines that she would no longer be in control of her medications. We would have to come up with a more creative solution for getting my mom her daily meds. Our solution was a medication lockbox. We would schedule a follow-up with a psychiatrist once she was discharged, and due to the anxiety my mom was feeling even with everyday life issues, we would need to find her a

Ch. 3 She is *Strong* for her mother...

therapist she could start seeing regularly. My mom would show me strength in dealing with so many personal issues publicly and facing some hard life truths.

It is one thing to have to deal with your deepest, darkest secrets in the comfort of your own mind and thoughts; it is a completely different scenario to deal with your deepest, darkest secrets with the people you love most. For me personally, before the incident, I had put my mom up on a pedestal without meaning to. I'd never considered that my mother was human, just like everyone else. I'd known my mother struggled with her health, but I had also watched her struggle and remain so strong day after day. Watching her come so close to death and then overcome such a dark incident, I knew God was not done with my mom here on earth. My mother would be the first to tell you she has not overcome her demons by herself; she gives me a lot of credit for always taking the time to care for her and care for the kids, especially by being the taxi driver to get everyone back and forth to their appointments. I have my strength because my mom taught me to never settle for anything less for myself.

After such a roller-coaster ride the last few years—after all that my dear mother had endured—she mustered up the strength to start and run her own ostomy group out of a local hospital here in our community. Talk about persevering! Her memory is still touch and go, and she has to make a lot of notes on her calendar to remember every detail of her week. Also, not being much of a group gal herself when it comes to attending groups to ask for support, the ostomy group was a huge project for my mom to take on. But she made the phone calls and did the legwork, and now, what do you know, she is using all her life experience to provide support for those who may be living under the same conditions and restrictions as her. As her daughter, I am so proud of my mom for continuing to do so much to keep herself going—for her to wake up and really use this second chance and do it right. Her weekly therapy has helped her deal with her anxiety and stay off of anxiety pills, and she has pushed through physical therapy to continue building up her strength on the left side of her body. She has found confidence through her work with the ostomy group, which has motivated her to publicly share her story with others many times. I find so much strength in the way she perseveres through so many hardships.

CHAPTER 4
She is *Strong* in her faith ...

Being strong in my faith is not something that comes easy to me. I ask lots of questions. I am constantly learning just how truly diverse a person's faith can be. It is something I still strive to educate and better myself in every day. I find the Bible absolutely fascinating—how can it be written by sinners like you and I so many centuries ago yet still show countless similarities to what you and I face in our lives today? It goes to show that our lives and our experiences are nothing new. There was trauma, heartache, envy, love, marriage, divorce, and betrayal long before you and I ever existed. So why do we feel like our faith is something we need to keep secret, or better yet, why do we feel like our faith is up for interpretation by others? The reality is, what we choose to believe in is our personal relationship with God. It's not about comparing my relationship with God to someone else's relationship with God.

I grew up in church, I was baptized as a baby, I had my first Holy Communion when I hit middle school, and I was confirmed. My mom made sure my brother and I didn't miss out on any opportunities to grow in our faith during our childhood. But when my mom's health issues really took a toll on her mind and body, it seemed our family's faith fell to the wayside. No one held me accountable for going to church. Most of the time, my mom was too sick to even make it to a traditional church service anymore. While I was commuting over an hour to CU Boulder and holding two jobs, church was nowhere in my weekend plans. I lived this way for years, paying no attention to my roots of faith. None of my friends were avid church attenders either, so it only felt right to go through the motions and live as though I was in control.

My first wedding brought back what I thought faith did for every young girl; you run back to it when big life events happen—good or bad events. My first husband and I were not faith based at all in our daily lives. Heck, we had never even been to a church service together or had a church to call home. But I was the only daughter my parents had, and I was the oldest child. Between my brother and I, I was the first to get married. Of course, money was an issue at the time, but my mom, dad, and grandparents made sure I had the fairy-tale wedding every little girl dreams of. My fiancé and I tried to do all the "right" things: we took marriage classes at the Catholic Church, did our daily wedding journals, and wrote our vows. All in all, we received the blessing of the priest so we could be married by the Catholic Church. This sounds so bad, but we basically checked off list after list to be sure we were doing this whole prewedding thing correctly.

My family threw us a huge Catholic wedding. I don't want to sound spoiled or ungrateful for this experience in my life, but I wish I had developed more of a backbone sooner. I wish I'd had a wise enough friend or family member to stop me or at least make me take a step back and truly think about what we were doing. Weddings like the one I had are not at all cheap. My family wrote huge checks and possibly got loans to pay for the big day. Looking back, everything about that day appeared to be faith based; it appeared to be perfect, in the sense that we took all the steps possible so our marriage would indeed be blessed. My wedding dress was straight out of a movie, with the long train and matching veil. My thinking was if my wedding looked like it needed to, then surely God would bless my marriage. But in reality, my heart was further away from God than it had ever been. Having the fancy church wedding did not keep my marriage going when our relationship hit hard times. Having the big church wedding did not save my marriage from ultimately ending in divorce. I learned strength in this season by realizing that there is so much more to the meaning of marriage, weddings, and faith in God than most people want to admit.

I continued to allow myself to stray further and further away from the church and my faith year after year. I am overwhelmed when I think of this season of my life and all the patience and grace God gave me. All the times God showed up for me when I couldn't even show up for myself. I am still in awe of God's power and love. It wasn't until I became a mother to my son and niece that I truly grasped the importance of having a relationship with God. The first death I experienced as a new mom was the death of a really good friend, a girl I'd gone to high school with. She was an amazing human being, and when she died, she left behind two precious babies. I was completely devastated for them. Blame it on my hormones as a new mom, since my son was only three months old, or call it God's perfect timing—either way, her passing affected me. Her passing caused me to think about my own life and the people in it.

Thank the Lord for sisters of faith...

I knew I needed to go back to church, but my childhood church was not at all equipped to handle small kids while I attended service. I will never forget my dear friend and neighbor who consistently invited my family to attend her church. She said I wouldn't be going alone, and I could sit by her. There was also a children's ministry where I could drop off my son and niece so I could truly enjoy an hour of service. I'd never been to church without my mom right beside me. I had never thought to seek God without my mom pushing me along. For the first time, I was seeking God because I needed him; I was struggling so hard in every area of my life, and I was seeking anything that might give me a glimpse of hope.

Finally, I agreed to try one church service with my neighbor. I convinced myself that if I didn't like it, then that would be that. The first Sunday at a new church, I was full of anxiety. I knew my mom suffered from anxiety, and while I had been experiencing this feeling more and more since becoming a new mom, I was determined to get a hold of myself. I got the kids successfully into the children's ministry, and then I found my neighbor and her family in the auditorium. The music started playing. It was beautiful music, and I had never seen any performance at a church like the one I witnessed that day. The lead singer had an amazing voice, and the lights changed colors with the beat of the drums. I'm sure it wasn't even two minutes before the tears started flowing and wouldn't stop. I was not at all expecting to have such a reaction just by walking in the doors and finding a seat.

One Sunday led to another Sunday, and before I knew what was happening, I started seeing changes within the kids, not just on Sundays but throughout the week. My niece was showing improvement in her temperament with my mom and stepdad and was finally showing signs of slowing down and not being so wild all the time. My son learned how to pray and what it meant to pray. Have you ever heard a one-and-a-half-year-old pray? It can bring a grown adult to tears. Both kids would run around the house, singing kids' songs they'd learned from Sunday school, which would bring back memories of what my brother and I used to do as children. We continued to go to church—just the three of us. I knew I was doing something bold in continuing to stand my ground with not only my husband, Shawn, but my mom and stepdad as well. None of them were against church, but at the time, none of them were equally as excited when Sunday came around and I would get the kids ready to go.

Ch. 4 She is *Strong* in her Faith...

After a few months of attending, I began to see the blessings church was providing for me. I can clearly remember my first Christmas at North Metro Church. It had been years since I'd attended church during the holidays. We were going through a series where our pastor and the entire staff at North Metro Church were putting on a play every Sunday in December. They were performing *A Christmas Carol*. If you haven't watched the musical of *A Christmas Carol*, I encourage you to find it online. The story line starts with a man named Ebenezer Scrooge; he's a grouchy man who is wealthy and successful. He chooses to live life very selfishly. To soften Ebenezer's heart, three ghosts visit him—the Ghost of Christmas Past, the Ghost of Christmas Present, and the Ghost of Christmas Yet-to-Come. When the Ghost of Christmas Past comes to see him, Ebenezer is reminded of a time when he was an innocent boy and the time when his insecurities began. Ebenezer had always picked money over friendships and relationships. Then came the Ghost of Christmas Present. Ebenezer was shown a man with his family. The man currently worked for Ebenezer, and the truth was that the man's young son would die unless the boy got proper medical treatment... but Ebenezer didn't care enough to help. Last was the Ghost of Christmas Yet-to-Come. This ghost was able to show Ebenezer the future he would have if he continued living in his selfish ways. He would die, and no one would really care, but of course they would show up to eat all the free food at his funeral service. The moral of *A Christmas Carol* is that life is not meant to be lived or to feel alone. Money can fill the void temporarily, but life means nothing when you have no one to do life with. *A Christmas Carol* brings to light why we need to cherish our friendships and family relationships.

I had seen *A Christmas Carol* so many times before I'd seen it performed at church, but I'd never caught the true message of why that story is so powerful. We had a week to reflect on each part of the play. I couldn't help but imagine if the Ghost of Christmas Past were to show up in my room—what would my ghost have to say to me? It was in this season at church I knew my life had to change. I needed to refocus on what kind of mother I wanted to be. I needed to buckle down and tackle all my hopes and dreams I had set for myself all those years ago. As time passed, my family started to see this church thing was not just a phase. I started volunteering in the children's ministry, and the kids were doing Vacation Bible School in the summer and kids' choir in the winter. I was living proof that change can happen when you let go and allow yourself to be changed.

Your actions speak louder than words...

My stepdad was the first person to take the leap of faith with me. It took him about a year or so of seeing my commitment to the church and getting the kids involved to realize that this was something worth being passionate about. God's mission for us is to go and make disciples (Matthew 28:19), and I quickly learned this idea was easier said than done. I say this because I have learned you can't force people to want what you want. You can't force people to choose to spend their time the way you do. After years of coming up with all sorts of reasons for why I could never go out and make disciples, I eventually realized I could make disciples just by setting an example in the way I lived my everyday life. Nothing fancy, nothing hard—just me remaining true and obedient to God, day in and day out, and my example of living would be enough. Please don't interpret this as me saying that I'm perfect and that I don't make mistakes, because—spoiler alert—I make mistakes all the time. But what makes this walk with God so incredible is that I can recognize my mistakes, and I repent; I will be the first to apologize when I am in the wrong, and I also work very hard at giving myself grace daily. When my stepdad started attending church with me, I remember being happy that finally someone in my immediate family was opening up to the idea that there was something more to life than just getting by. Once I figured out he was just as serious about

Ch. 4 She is *Strong* in her Faith...

attending church as I was, and he was getting the help he needed to conquer his own demons, I got to sit back and truly thank God for showing me what it felt like to live out his mission of making disciples. I showed strength in my faith to live and let go, truly letting God take control of my life.

In May 2014, Shawn and I finally committed to the married life. Since I had been married before, I didn't think it would be appropriate for us to have a big wedding, nor is my husband fond of crowds, so the idea of a big wedding didn't amuse him either. My husband, coming from a family of outdoorsmen, thought our wedding would be perfect at his buddy's parents' house. They had some land and a nice shop, which, if you didn't know any better, looked like a barn. We would borrow hay bales for our guests to sit on. This was going to be a low-key wedding, with no traditional pastor, groomsmen, or bridesmaids. My dad had walked me down the aisle once, and this time, since our son was one year old and walking, he would be the one to walk me down the aisle (pure bliss). We would have our closest family and friends attend our special evening, and my son's godfather would be the one to marry us. It couldn't have gone any better. The night was complete with a DJ and a barbecue dinner. It was absolutely perfect! Completely a different setup from my first wedding, and way less pressure.

My husband had never been the type to not believe in God. He just has questions—sometimes, questions I cannot answer for him. Although our wedding and marriage did not appear to be faith based on the outside because we were not in a church and we did not have a traditional pastor do our ceremony, that did not make our wedding any less meaningful. In the end, he and I vowed to each other and to our families—in sickness and in health, for richer or for poorer, we said, "I do," for the simple fact that we will fight for our family.

Amazing people come into your life when you choose to share your faith with others. I'd never pictured myself being able to reference my favorite Bible stories or verses in conversations before. I'd never pictured myself being a mother and having a child who cries because he wants me to read one more Bible story from his kids' Bible before bedtime. My husband has even opened up more to the idea of church and figuring out where he stands in his faith. We joined a marrieds' group at church within the past year, and while I had hesitation about even joining the group in the first place, to my surprise, week after week, the couples that show up are looking for a place to belong. We have a rather big group, as there are about nine couples in total, but from what we share with each other and what we pray about with each other, it's clear that this group is a safe zone. No one is judged because their views and ideas differ from other couples'. We are not judged for how we choose to raise our kids, what schools they go to, or how much money we make or don't make. It is truly a group of other married couples looking to belong—looking to build healthy, positive relationships outside of the church walls. My husband, who hates being in large crowds and is very much an introvert, enjoys going to our weekly marrieds' group. It's amazing to hear him converse and offer knowledge to our new friends.

I do think that in my lifetime, the work we will be most known for will be the work we choose to do in our involvement with the church, and although that is not where we are just yet, I know God is planting that seed in my husband and I now. Disciples come when you least expect it. My husband quit an HVAC career of twenty years. The job my husband had had the last seven years did not fulfill him anymore. Instead, it made him angry, agitated, and short-tempered. I was convinced if my husband stayed at his job, he would ultimately hurt his health, and although that job provided our family with financial security, I, as a wife, was not willing to risk my husband's life for a job any longer. We are still in a season of uncertainty, and while interview after interview keep falling through for him, I am certain God has a much bigger plan for him than we can even think up on our own.

Ch. 4 She is *Strong* in her Faith...

I have not always been so dedicated in my faith journey, as I am not a girl who does well with confrontation. I tend to talk about my faith with people I know are like minded and not prone to challenge my thoughts or ideas regarding what I believe in. As I write my thoughts out on paper, I know it sounds cowardly, but it's true. My faith journey wouldn't be where it is today if I didn't allow myself to be challenged in my thinking about God and the Bible. I am also a visual learner, and taking a job at a children's hospital added some perspective to my beliefs. Visiting a children's hospital, when you walk in the doors, you feel and see immediately why places like this are worthy of being supported not only financially, but spiritually as well.

Working at a children's hospital and helping families firsthand during some of the worst times of their lives will bring a person to their knees, thanking God for all the small things we take for granted. While I always dreamed of being a nurse, I also know I am not at all equipped to deal with the blood and guts that arise during emergencies. Instead, my role at the hospital is to educate families about the various insurance programs that exist to help families ease the heavy burdens of financial debt that may accrue while their child is ill. My expertise is in government programs such as Medicaid, low-income Medicaid, Child Health Plan Plus, Medicaid Buy-In, and Medicaid waivers, just to name a few. I also help families apply for government assistance such as the Colorado Indigent Care Program and our hospital program, also known as the charity program. In a role like mine, I have very limited time to listen to families about the needs of their children, educate each family on what programs I feel would benefit their family, and then help them complete the lengthy applications and get them turned in to the correct offices for processing. Usually, I am doing these exact things for a family that is under an unbelievable amount of stress and most likely not even wanting to be in my office to handle such tasks. It's in the times with these families that I get to see all stages of denial and acceptance play out. It's times like these—when I start by having an off morning, feeling sorry for myself—that I am quickly reminded there is always someone who has it so much worse than I do. It's times like this when I am thankful I found my faith again so I can pray with a family if that's what they need to make it another hour before getting a test result or to leave the hospital for the last time without their child next to them.

My faith was not at all a job requirement, nor do these situations happen every day. But I can tell you that when it does happen, when I can sense a family is truly looking for hope, and I happen to be that contact, being confident in my faith is a reassurance that this is what I am here for. Having the strength to pray for someone who may be a stranger to me—that alone may cause someone to reconsider what faith means to them. My faith was not reignited solely by my own doing; if you remember, I had a friend, who was also my neighbor, gently extend an invitation for me to try her church, week after week. Discipleship comes when you least expect it, and transformation won't happen by being the pushy churchgoer or by always being right in your beliefs. Transformation happens because you allow people to come to their faith on their terms and for no other reason than they are seeking something more for their lives. It is possible to find such a freedom and love for the job you choose to be at day after day, and I am living proof of that.

I share these stories of my faith to inspire those who maybe feeling lost like I was, or those who let the weight of everyday stress fall on their shoulders. I can relate because of the chains I allowed to be placed on me when I lived life that way, lost and guided by stress. It was exhausting, and looking back, I was not truly living in those days. I was just getting by the best way I knew how. God knows our wants and needs even before we ourselves can recognize what they are. I sought God's words and wisdom in a time of my life when I was broken, truly broken. God's word tell us in 1 Peter 5:7, "Cast all your anxiety on him because he cares for you." This idea may take you some time to work through, but in the times of my life where anxiety took over my soul and filled my mind with doubt, being

Ch. 4 She is *Strong* in her Faith...

able to hand those burdens over to God felt amazing. Heck, I'm still here writing about it and praising his name. My life will forever be changed because I allowed my faith to guide me every day; faith gives me hope for a better tomorrow.

CHAPTER 5
She is *Strong* for others . . .

It takes a special kind of bravery to put yourself out in the world—to share your story with complete strangers. But if I have learned anything from "life" as we know it, I've learned that my story may offer healing to someone else's heartache. I am just one person in this big ole world, and encouraging others is not always easy. Encouraging others is hard work; sometimes, the people you want to encourage most don't want you to encourage them at all. Am I right? Encouraging others is challenging because, quite frankly, you don't feel qualified enough. I have felt this way many times in my life. Something that has worked to keep me motivated and keep me on the mission to encourage others is realizing this life I have been given is not about *me*—that's right, when I encourage others well, it is because I've chosen to realize the bigger picture; this life is not about me. Okay, yes, to some extent it is healthy to be selfish sometimes, and I will write all about that topic on its own. But truly, reader, life is not meant to be lived selfishly or to feel alone. I encourage others every chance I get. I will buy my friend flowers when I know she is having a tough week. I will get involved with the Facebook groups of women who, a few times a year, will make care packages for one another, just for the mere reason that it's nice to receive a true surprise once in a while. Another way I encourage that costs nothing is through writing reviews. Reviews for anything, such as my Uber driver, my gym trainer, and my Audible audiobooks. I have a friend who is absolutely great at checking in on me randomly. She will send sweet messages that say "Good morning! Praying for you guys," and I love her for that. She will never know how much I have truly needed to hear her words on a particular day. Encouraging others is hard; it does take practice and may seem to some like kissing ass!

Honestly, a simple text, the coffee date you kept on the calendar for weeks, that chat in the lunchroom, or the one hour you spent at the park with a friend or a stranger—dig for ways you can encourage people in your circle. Heck, maybe it's your spouse who needs the encouragement. I know my spouse has been going through a season of frustration, and while I cannot fix his situation, with God's help, I can encourage a good mood; I can encourage him to have a positive attitude about our current situation, the best way I know how.

People notice when you show up for them. People also notice when you show up for yourself. What that looks like for me is following through with my online Bible study group, showing up for my disabled mom to get her to a doctor's appointment, and do her weekly medications and showing up for my coworkers, even when, by golly, I truly just feel like I need to take a day off. My husband sees me lead by example daily; this has been encouraging to him. I didn't know this was the case until he left me a note saying so before he went on a hunting trip. Any of you ladies or men know what encouraging notes from your spouse or anyone close to you can do to your heart?! Mine just about exploded! I cried and cried. Happy tears, of course, because all along, I was just doing my thing, and it is a blessing to know my husband, in a season of figuring out his "why" in life, has noticed me taking action and taking a stand for my life.

Finding your "why" in life means finding what gets you moving every day. What make you tick and want to achieve more greatness day after day? My number one answer is my family. They deserve me

Ch. 5 She is *Strong* for others...

being the best mama, wife, daughter, friend, etc. I mentioned that my husband is still in the process of figuring out his "why" because this past year, he was so hard on himself. He felt like a failure when it came to his career, when it came to supporting his family, and there was a moment where I, his wife, was worried about where his mental state was going and insisted he start therapy. When people tend to not set individual goals for themselves and let their identities get wrapped up in a career path, destruction happens. An easy example I can think of is when I say "I work as a financial counselor" rather than saying "I am a financial counselor." I may be a financial counselor, but my title does not define me. Instead when I say, I work as a financial counselor; I get to choose every day to help families who are underinsured or not insured at all.

Being strong for others is still something I work on day after day, and for me, it involves setting boundaries. It is far too easy to get entirely wrapped up in someone else's bad situation, and before I know it, their bad situation has now become my problem. Relationships have been ruined because of my lack in setting boundaries for myself at the get-go. When we bought our house seven years ago, it wasn't long before my husband and I started opening our home to let people stay with us. We weren't always in agreement, but we would never let any of our family members go homeless. By offering our help, not necessarily with money but by offering a place to stay instead, we could help them get on their feet. Most of the time, that meant we had to front the bill for higher electric and gas bills as well as grocery bills, since there were more people to feed. Just everyday household bills also went up because there were more bodies in our home day to day. A few years ago, my younger brother and his family were in a position where they too needed a change and a chance to save money and get on their feet. Since it was my brother, of course I said yes, and being a new auntie, I was stoked I would get to see my nephews daily. This was not going to be a small move for Mark and his family, as they had to move from another state to Colorado. Our home was not necessarily huge, so for their family of six and my family of three, we had to get creative to prepare beds for everyone to sleep in. We turned our front room into a bedroom for the teenager, we had my toddler son and their toddler son share a bedroom, and then my brother, his wife, and their babies would share a room with Pack 'n Plays side by side. It was a tight squeeze, but we all made it work. The day my brother and his family arrived, I was so excited! I had not lived in the same state as my brother in over ten years. I was ready to start building a relationship with my sister-in-law, as our relationship had previously only consisted of short talks on the phone and on Facebook. I made sure the rooms were stocked with everything the kids might need: clothes, diapers, hangers, dressers, lights—seriously, all the essentials. Things went well in the beginning, and everyone seemed to be adjusting well and pitching in with all the household chores.

As the older sister, I have always been protective, not only of my mom but of my brother as well, and rightfully so—when we were children, it was my job to fill in as a parent for Mark when both my parents were either sick or too busy with their lives to know where us kids and our feelings truly stood.

As the days turned into months, I witnessed just how much my brother and his family struggled, and it broke my heart. They were fighting demons in their family life that I had never witnessed before, nor had my brother spoken about them on the phone during our weekly talks. I was new in my faith, and seeing what church had done in my life offered up an idea. I knew my brother had been taking his own kids to service where they'd previously lived, but I'd never been the pushy church family member, so even extending such an offer to my brother and his family was out of my comfort zone. They attended with me, though we were like a big Brady Bunch family when we pulled into the church parking lot. I was not at all sure how I alone could fix my brother and his family's brokenness all by myself, but I knew God alone had worked to fix

Ch. 5 She is *Strong* for others...

my heart and my heartache, so why couldn't he do the same for my brother's family?

More time went by, and in the close quarters of our families living together, our different parenting styles were starting to wear thin on all of us adults in the home. The teenager was getting into more trouble at her high school, being bullied by teen girls, and dealing with all the things high school girls deal with regarding boys. I still had not seen my brother and his wife make any headway in getting on their own two feet. I became angry about the entire situation. Personally, I was frustrated and disappointed. My brother and I had been taught so many life lessons as children on how to deal with hard situations and, more importantly, on how to make an epic comeback from hard life lessons. My husband, God bless him, talked me off the ledge of a family fight more times in a day than I would like to admit. There I was, wanting to help my brother and his family, fix all their problems, and then send them on their merry way to independence. In my mind, none of that should have been too hard to achieve, but instead of having an epic comeback story, my brother and I had an epic family fight. I don't know about you, but fighting was not something my brother and I did much, even as kids; I was always his protector, and I always kept him out of harm's way or gave him money when he was short. He was my baby brother, and I loved him dearly! The one person who was basically programmed to love me forever now doesn't even acknowledge me.

Looking back now in the calm after the storm, I realize that my brother and I should have thought more about living with each another but also adding our spouses and kids into the mix, we set up false expectations of one another. I thought my brother ran his household a certain way—I thought that because of our experiences and what we had been through as kids, he was a stronger person. All the expectations I came up with in my head were high-level expectations, ones I hold myself accountable to, and my brother did not come close to any of them. It would take me reading a lot of scripture, praying with others, and sharing my story to realize that being strong for others does not mean solving all their life problems. Being strong for others could simply be providing an ear for them to vent to or a gentle hug and a shoulder for them to cry on.

Lots of tears have been shed, words have been said that can never be taken back, and now there are cousins who will grow up possibly not knowing one another, but my "why" in life has always had me standing up for the truth—to speak truth even when the truth is difficult to hear.

For the longest time, I would not have called this a blessing, but rather more of a curse. When I am passionate about something, or when I see a family member being mistreated, used, or abused, it pains my heart to just stay out of it. Especially when I see potential in a situation to make things better. My "why" motivation and the leadership inside of me prompts me to want to fix all the problems—if only *they* would listen. Has anyone felt this way before? Maybe you have witnessed a family member or friend struggling with something you fought years before—perhaps you already know the outcome, but they just won't give you the time of day to help them.

I am here to tell you that once you understand your "why" in life, you are able to understand why you respond the way you do to certain topics. My "why" causes me to want to fix everything, but in reality, I am not God and do not hold that power. I am not powerful enough to make everyone listen to me. So in understanding my "why," I am also able to figure out my triggers and why "be slow to anger" is such an important scripture for me to live by. Realizing it's okay to let people fail is also significant—yes, I said it, and let me say it again! It is okay to let people fail! When you are constantly fixing every situation for your loved ones, they become dependent and needy. They will never learn for themselves how to succeed if you don't allow them the opportunity to fail, myself included in this. God allows the heart to heal in time, and while I

Ch. 5 She is *Strong* for others...

will always love my brother and his kids, right now, in this season, I have learned it is best for me to love them from afar.

Stepping out of your comfort zone...

Community service work has always been something my mom trained us kids to be a part of and something I learned about from an early age. (Thank you, Girl Scouts.) While I didn't always enjoy volunteering at my local animal shelter, it was helpful to the business and the animals I got to play with. Community service work can be time consuming and almost feel daunting when you serve in places that you don't have a general interest in serving, and it wasn't until I was an adult that I truly figured this out.

Even before I worked at the children's hospital, I always envisioned helping their hospital in some way, and I did, either through donating money during their Radio-Thon with 105.9, a local morning show here in Colorado, or choosing to make a care package for sick cancer patients who would be spending the holidays in the hospital. It wasn't till I worked for the children's hospital that I realized the extent of what volunteering meant and why holding fundraisers for the hospital was so important. Being able to not only be a team member but to volunteer my time at events such as A Taste of Colorado or a Denver Broncos game speaks volumes, not only to the people who know me but to families who spend days, months, and sometimes years coming to the facility.

My son is in elementary school now—anyone else who has young children in elementary school knows there are a lot of fundraisers, movie nights, and holiday events that the PTO members put on for the kids. In order for these events to be successful, volunteers are needed. While I can't always help with every event, I have realized the need to serve in my child's school and make it a priority to volunteer in the classroom and at PTO events. Parents or grandparents who have kids in grade school, I encourage you to reach out to your local PTO team, even if that means that only a few times during the school year, you giving them your time—even for just a few hours will make all the difference, especially to the men and women who take the time and effort to plan these events.

Serving in my community doesn't only happen through the children's hospital or my child's school, but also in my local church. When I finally made the decision to accept Christ back into my life, I went all in, and that meant volunteering in the children's ministry. I have young kids myself, and getting creative in order to serve while also not keeping my kids in class for too long (mom guilt is real) meant I would sacrifice going to church service one Sunday a month to serve, and then I would catch up on the sermon once it was posted online.

In my early walk with faith, while I was reconnecting with the church, it took a lot out of me to get myself and the kids ready Sunday after Sunday to do our "church thing," and while most Sundays it would have been easier to say, "Forget it, let's miss service today and stay in our jammies," I would think of all the times God had shown up for me. Training my mind to think about God this way changed my life; if God could show up for me day after day and love me for all that I am, why am I complaining about showing up for him and serving his people on Sundays? God showed me strength in scripture about how loving on others was necessary, not only for my own heart but for the families I served as well.

It wasn't until I created my own personal blog that I realized the full power my words and writing could have on people. In the first month and a half of having my blog site, I had people reading my blog from all over the world. Places such as India, Ireland, and Australia—places my little ole mind can only dream of visiting one day. I quickly realized there was a great need for someone who can generate inspiring content—someone who is willing to be raw, real, and humble at the expense of sharing pieces of my heart. Blogging is nothing new, but this scene was new to me, and getting Facebook messages from complete strangers telling me they could relate or that my blog provides them hope to carry on to the next day was inspiring in itself.

Not all my posts offer faith content, because, for one, I am human, and some days it's completely okay not to be pushy about all the things the good Lord has been doing in my life. I have also learned that while I can do all things through Christ who strengthens me, I need to give myself some credit too. I work hard; I don't expect any of God's gifts to just come to me.

I realized I needed to fully understand my "why" and the mission behind my "why." God's word is effective not only in what we say but in how we choose to live out his word, meaning I can't just tell you, my readers, that I am a godly woman, and you need to take my word for it. I would get so much hate mail if I did that. Instead, I share my life experiences, share my testimony with you all, and have you visualize all the reasons why I no longer say, "It was just a coincidence"—because, you guys, the works of the Lord are not at all coincidences.

Reading back through some of my daily blog posts and the words I used to describe my busy life, I see that there is no way I alone—physically or emotionally—could have gotten through all those hard days. While I was by my mom's side through all her health struggles when I was a young child, I was not alone. Through the anger and resentment I felt in my failed marriage, I was not alone. Watching my mom lifeless on the living room floor, I was not alone. Walking into a new church as an adult, I was not alone.

I truly think my blog is so successful with believers and nonbelievers for the simple fact that my writing and my experiences help others see hope, no matter how bad your situation may seem. I also try to challenge my readers about the topics I am writing about, whether that be encouraging others, writing gratitude, paying it forward, or getting you to move your body. I write out challenges for my readers, who, to some extent, may need that kick-in-the-butt kind of message. I am learning how to be strong when it comes to God providing a platform such as a blog or social media, and I'm learning how effective it can be in changing the way people communicate with and educate one another.

Give grace...

I enjoy going to conferences and listening to keynote speakers. I was recently able to see Paul Schmidt, and the audience was asked to think about the first time or maybe the last time we'd stepped up for ourselves or someone else. He asked, "How did that experience make you feel? Did you catch yourself being able to step up a second time?"

Recently, I had to stick up for someone I know. I'd watched this person be talked to negatively day after day, given negative looks, and gossiped about among mutual friends. Finally, enough was enough, and although I don't like being involved in confrontation, I stepped up. Not because I was asked to step up, but because I believe people need to be treated as equals. People need to be valued, loved, and praised for all their talents. As Paul Schmidt said, this idea will take lots of practice, but the more situations we encounter where we can step up instead of stepping back, the more these so-called difficult conversations can be done successfully.

Most of the time, the people who create difficult situations for everyone are struggling with their own insecurities or problems, and they tend to take out their frustrations on the ones they love the most—or worse, on complete strangers. But what we need to recognize is no two people are the same; we won't all do the same things or like the same things, but that doesn't give anyone the right to put others down because they don't believe what you do or operate the way you do. Sticking up for this person made me feel good, and it solved a problem that had been likely to escalate.

Ch. 5 She is *Strong* for others...

Paul Schmidt also had us think about our list of things we suck at—yes, I know! He said to make a list of the things we suck at and, after writing them down, share this list with the people you interact with daily: family, friends, and coworkers. By doing this, we can help others learn more about us, and this allows us each to take ownership of the things we suck at. It may even provide a little motivation to do better and hold ourselves accountable for our areas of improvement. The list may seem a little harsh, but as Paul told us about his experience in sharing his list with his employees, he explained that it had pleasantly surprised him. Everyone had nodded in agreement that his list was indeed accurate, and everyone had had a little laugh from his honesty. Laughter can be therapeutic, and in the heat of a disagreement, a good laugh can help lighten the mood. For myself, laughter causes me to not take myself so seriously. I found both of Paul Schmidt's ideas very inspirational and even shared them on my blog page right after the conference. I have learned that being strong for others means stepping up in a world that has me so quickly wanting to step down.

I am only one person; I am only in control of my emotions and no one else's. I am not this powerful being that has control over others and how they feel about me, whether those be good or bad feelings. If others are frustrated with me or just cannot resonate with me, then so be it—how they express themselves is completely up to them. But I am no longer holding myself responsible for pleasing everyone.

Have you ever wondered why people may not resonate with you? Maybe to some extent, they are jealous of the life you live. Maybe they want the same relationships with people that you are able to generate. Whatever the reason, it seems to me the people we tend not to resonate with are the ones we tiptoe around the most. I am learning this firsthand. I have always called myself the "doer," meaning I get shit done when it needs to be done. I can't stand it when people beat around the bush; we will get more accomplished if you are straight with me in your expectations. Because I am a doer, I also tend to be more productive in my day-to-day activities. As I have said before, I consider myself a master of juggling 101 things on my daily to-do list. In saying that, I also know when it's appropriate to ask others for help. I'm not shy in that regard. But personally, when I feel burned, used, or not appreciated for things I go out of my way to do for people, I choose to walk away, take it as lesson learned, and go on with life. I won't soak in all the what-ifs and wonder how I could fix that relationship. Because, if I am being honest, we don't grow as individuals by constantly referring to the past. If I strive to be a better me than I was yesterday, this is only going to happen 100 percent when I learn and accept that in this life, I am not going to please everyone and meet their so-called expectations they have set for me.

What does it look like in your life to give grace? For me personally, I have really had to practice this concept with my son, at my job, and with my family. Giving someone grace is not about letting them win—to me, giving grace to someone is allowing your mind to open up to a new way of thinking and not attacking the other person for their way of thinking. Instead, ponder their words a bit and allow yourself to process and not speak with hate on your tongue.

Giving grace does not always have to be something you do for others either. There are many times I have to practice giving grace to myself, to not allow my mind to be so hard on my physical body. Giving grace to ourselves is oftentimes easier said than done and, at times, takes a lot of practice to achieve results. What I have found to be rather interesting is the correlation between giving grace to ourselves and giving grace to others. The two seem to go hand in hand, and once you work hard to give grace to yourself, it seems—or at least for me—that giving grace to others is not such an impossible task.

CHAPTER 6
She is *Strong* in her health . . .

My relationship with food has not always been healthy. I was extremely active in sports when I was a child and never struggled with being overweight, but my relationship with food was never something I was proud of. Remember, I was the child who was eating pizza for breakfast at my dad's pizzeria most weekend mornings. My maternal grandpa, Tony, always called me his "cow," not to be mean, but because this girl could eat. That nickname hurt my feelings as a young child, but when he passed away while I was in my twenties, I realized just how much I missed his voice and the cow comments.

In high school, my relationship with food didn't get any better. I got lunch money from my parents, and so many lunch hours were spent at our local Wendy's, Subway, Taco Bell, and McDonald's. Fast food would feed my soul and provide comfort when my life as a teenager became overwhelming and stressful. While I always appeared to be healthy and fit, it wasn't until my freshman year of college that my metabolism failed me, and freshman fifteen hit me with a vengeance.

Freshman fifteen is just a myth, right? I'd always believed that this idea was indeed made up to scare young girls, but I am living proof it can and will happen when you are not taking care of your body. I don't remember what the numbers on the scale were when I started my first year of college versus when I ended my first year of college, but I know that by the end of my first year of college, boy did those skinny jeans no longer go over my thighs. I had all intentions of playing tennis for CU Boulder—tennis was a sport I'd played from a young age. It was a sport I was good at and a sport that helped keep my mind sharp. But the day I went to the CU Boulder tennis tryouts, I couldn't even get myself to go out on the courts. This was the first time I remember letting fear truly take over and letting all the lies and negative thoughts speak to my soul. I walked away from that opportunity feeling like I was not good enough and, in the end, not trying out for the team.

I had never been the girl who backed down from a challenge, but in that season of my life, I was sure all my training had not prepared me to play tennis for a college team. I would go from being very active in high school with cheerleading, dancing, swimming, and playing tennis to doing absolutely no sports whatsoever. This type of shock to my body caused my body to put on weight very quickly.

I have rejection issues—like most, it's not something I openly talk about, because in all reality, who wants to be in a conversation with someone who is having a pity party for themselves? But I feel like this topic is important and one that needs to be addressed, because we only get stronger as individuals when we choose to take risks and when we recognize what it is in our lives that we need to fix. For me, fear of rejection persists because I never feel qualified enough to talk, even on a subject I have spent a lot of time researching. I am always the one second-guessing myself. I never want to get my facts wrong, nor do I want to write about a subject that people have no interest in reading. Those negative thoughts and

Ch. 6 She is *Strong* in her health...

perceptions hold me back at times, and trying out for the tennis team in college was one of those times.

Self-doubt has also occurred while writing this book, not because I am having a hard time writing, but because I wonder, "What will people think?" What I do know is I am very much aware of what I am doing, and I will overcome my fear of rejection. I am writing a book through my trials, even if my story is still not finished. Thank you to Rachel Hollis for these words that repeat in my mind: "What other people think of me is none of my business." See, reader, my fear of rejection is very real! I struggle with my thoughts just like most of you do. But in my struggle, I refuse to give up or let my fears win. I refuse to give up on my dreams. Even if my book helps just one person, then that's a win. My prayer for all of us is to give ourselves some grace when it comes to tackling the unknowns. Our fears are not our burdens to keep; give them up to the Lord. Maybe you have one fear, or maybe you're like me and have multiple fears. Whatever it is, don't make the mistake I made in letting fear run your life. I became strong in my health because I no longer let fear have a voice.

The weight gain continued even when I married my first husband. The condo we purchased even had a little gym with basic workout equipment that I did not even consider using when we first bought our place. In that season of my life, I was sure that my lifestyle was what "adulting" looked and felt like. But after multiple years of living this way, neglecting my self-image, I became lonely, sad, and very depressed. Call this a feel-bad-for-myself moment, but I can clearly remember one late night—I was awake and couldn't sleep, and you know what came on the screen? A Beachbody infomercial with fit ladies telling me all the reasons why I needed the nine-DVD box set and how I could do these workouts all in the comfort of my own home. I thought, "Wait! No one would have to see me struggling to work out! Great!"

I called the number on the screen, I requested the Express Mail option, and I set up monthly installment payments to pay off what I'm sure now was over five hundred dollars (Dave Ramsey would kill me for such an impulsive purchase). But I did it and very excitedly waited for the mail the next few days. My order came on time, and while I was excited to start such a heavy task, my husband at the time was not at all supportive. I heard it all—I was beautiful the way I was, with or without the added weight. He was sure this would only be a phase and I would give up within a week or so, because who had time to diet anyway? But I started the program without his support; I was determined to be strong for myself. I didn't want to shop for size eighteen jeans ever again!

Anybody who has done the Beachbody workouts can see why those ladies are so fit, because the videos can go forever and ever. For someone who had not worked out in over five years, starting out with a forty-five-minute workout or the one-hour video was too intimidating. Then, in the back of my DVD collection, I found a twenty-minute workout. I am sure now it was meant as a pre-workout warm-up, but when I realized I was not cut out for the other videos, that twenty-minute workout became my go-to video daily. I stuck with the Beachbody video till I got down to a comfortable size twelve. I am not sure many people even noticed my weight loss, as I learned to wear my weight well, or so I thought.

Life continued, divorce came about with my husband, and continued depression and life fails would prove to be the best weight-loss remedy, and that didn't take much effort at all. I could now get into size ten jeans. Woot woot! A group of coworkers and I considered joining a 24 Hour Fitness, where we could take spin classes, Zumba, and swimming to work on our figures. Along with our memberships, we would get a few free one-on-ones with a gym trainer too—basically, a hot trainer would try to show my girlfriends and I some techniques that we cared absolutely nothing about because we were too gaga for how good-looking our trainer was. After getting this gym membership, I grew to love the Zumba classes. I had always been a good dancer. Use dancing to get in my exercise and fitness? I was sold. Going to class and making a fool out of how my body didn't move like my instructors did made the workouts fun and always made me laugh. I never felt like I was in class for a full hour.

At this point in my life, I realized I needed to make fitness a priority, but I continued to eat all the wrong foods. Everyone loves good ole McDonald's or Wendy's french fries, and although I was working out, I was still missing a vital piece of the puzzle to truly be successful in managing my health. I read somewhere that success can be compared to sitting at the top of a whole bunch of failed attempts, and I can relate with that idea.

For years, I was off and on with working on my fitness and myself. When I got pregnant, I remember thinking I would be the pregnant mama who was literally all belly and didn't gain all the extra baby weight. Oh, precious old self, you make me laugh! That thought lasted an entire week before pregnancy cravings hit me out of left field, and when the cravings came on—oh boy! The only thing that could satisfy me was a quick fast-food drive-through or a good bowl of cereal to get it over with. My pregnancy proved to be rather hard, not only with the way I saw myself in the mirror, but also with my mindset in general.

Don't get me wrong, I was super excited about being a new mama but not equally excited that I was forever swollen, and watching the scale climb to over two hundred pounds was depressing. I know I am not alone when I write out these words, and a part of me feels guilty for even complaining about something so simple as weight gain, especially because I know some of you reading this may struggle with infertility and would go through great lengths to even be able to carry a child. But I also can't dismiss those thoughts I once had about myself and how I felt during my pregnancy journey. What I am sure of now is I was not in the best shape prebaby; I did not prepare myself for what pregnancy actually was or should be like. The weak core I had prebaby would become even weaker, adding on nine months of carrying a child and not doing any exercises at all. When I was pregnant, I even complained about walking (oh, I hear all the sighs—poor me). But, you guys, I am here to say that all I experienced prebaby and during pregnancy was my fault. I could have done a much better job preparing myself and my mindset for such a life-changing event. Instead I went into it thinking, "Oh, this is just how it is. No fun, and let's just sit it out; let's truly see just how big I can get."

Urijah Gage was born, and while I loved him more than anything in the world, it hit me almost immediately that I'd just done something that would change my body forever. I had justified my big belly because, of course, there had been a baby inside of it that needed to grow healthy and strong to enter this world. But when Urijah came, and my belly was now a saggy mess with stretch marks all over, I truly felt it would take more than a miracle to get my old body back—you know, the body that I had been trying to change for years before pregnancy. I'd struggled with my health then, and having a baby and sagging skin made me truly realize I knew nothing about how to get healthy or how to even maintain good health.

I did what I thought every new mom did; I bought "magic" pills, meal replacement drinks, and so much more. When those didn't give me instant results, I moved on to the next new fad, the next new body oil treatments, wraps—you name it, and I am sure I tried it. All these things guaranteed me what I wanted, which were *results*. I am sad to admit this, but I lived this way, looking for my quick fix, for far too long. I wouldn't grasp a healthy lifestyle or workout regimen till I found a local trainer who was holding workouts at a park near my house. I'd been hearing all the crazed reviews, and people had told me they were hard workouts, but so many people were seeing crazy results. Story after story was being told on social media. The trainer's program grew so rapidly from exercises at the park to him renting a small but decent space to hold classes. So what did I have to lose?

Ch. 6 She is *Strong* in her health...

Mom guilt again is a real thing. For those reading this, moms getting involved in anything outside of the home that doesn't involve the kids causes so much guilt, and I am not even sure why. I'm lucky that my current husband, who is my son's dad, is amazingly supportive at really anything I decide to venture into. I'm sure he was tired of hearing me moan and groan. I'm sure he was tired of hearing me complain about how tired I was all day every day. Either way, he supported my fitness journey financially and emotionally; he was all in when it came to helping out with the kids and making healthy meals.

My first class at HIITBox was so hard! I was not at all comfortable in my newly bought workout clothes. I wasn't even convinced I could stick to the program for long, so I refused to buy a sports bra or proper tennis shoes. After burning through three Walmart bras and literally popping a hole in my tennis shoes, I finally figured out this wasn't a phase, and I wouldn't be stopping the program anytime soon. HIITBox classes turned into strength classes (lifting weights) and yoga, which was a huge deal for me, because if you knew me at all, I would have been the first to say I was not cut out for yoga or that I was too fast-paced for yoga. Turns out, I was really good at giving myself all the excuses for why yoga was not for me.

My first yoga class was a yoga flow class. It moved at a slightly faster pace than traditional yoga, and I liked that, but the positions were tough. I still have not mastered any of them. I was so naive about how much you actually sweat in yoga; I would be covered and dripping with sweat by the end of class. One class led to another at HIITBox, and I started seeing my body change. My skin was tightening in areas I had not seen tighten in years. I wasn't even worried so much about the number on the scale anymore; it was more about figuring out that in general, I was feeling so much better about myself and my health. Before HIITBox, I had really been struggling with chronic stomach issues. I'd had my gallbladder surgically removed. I had been on IBS medication and stomach spasm medication, and I couldn't figure out what the heck my problem was. I was only thirty and having tests done that people in their seventies were having done.

Once I found HIITBox, and once the weight started coming off, all the routine doctors' appointments slowed down. I was able to get off all the prescribed medications and manage my health strictly through diet and exercise. I don't want to say exercise and diet alone can cure everyone, but in my case, this was my body's way of telling me I could no longer keep feeding myself harmful foods. Going to HIITBox three to four times a week and sometimes needing to bring the kids due to scheduling conflicts with my husband's job started changing our family dynamic. Soon, my son and my niece were seeing firsthand what it takes to take care of yourself—what it takes for me to be strong for myself so I can continue to take care of them and be strong for everyone else.

I have a family video of my four-year-old son wanting to be like mommy, doing his push-ups. He lets out a huge fart, and we start laughing hysterically, because we all know lots of running or push-ups cause gas. Ultimately, I was a being a role model to these kids and teaching them about fitness even before I really understood that little eyes were indeed watching and learning from how I managed stress and self-care.

Do you fill your own cup . . . ?

There is a misconception when someone talks about health and only refers to taking care of your health as far as getting the right amount of exercise per day or per week. It wasn't until recently that I discovered that being strong in my health meant more than moving my body or eating the right foods; it also comes in the form of music I listen to, books I read or listen to, and even the people I choose to spend my time with. All of these things have contributed to me actively working on being strong in my health. I am a huge book nerd; I was when I was a little girl, and somewhere along the path of growing up, I quit making time to read books for pleasure. Chalk it up to me being a thirteen-year-long college student and constantly having a new textbook to read or a test to study for, but I quit reading for pleasure. Since college graduation in October 2017, reading for pleasure is something I have excitedly gotten back into. I read all the time, about anything and everything. I am big into reading memoirs from big and not-so-big authors. I enjoy reading about personal development and how most personal development coaches had to hit rock bottom in order to make it to the top. I also find scripture and all the stories in the Bible fascinating—sometimes to the degree of overwhelming, especially when I start to think that in my lifetime, I will never fully understand all the scriptures and their true meanings. I enjoy digging into Bible studies and going line by line, page by page, to fully understand the message written within that part of the book. I get asked all the time, how on earth do I make time to read, run a blog, write a book, and participate in a Bible study? My answer is simple: doing these things fills my cup, and when I have a full cup, my overall health and stress levels are down.

When I have a full cup, I am not so tired and can continue to be a good wife, a good mom, a good daughter, a good friend, etc. If you have never heard of the term, "Fill your own cup," that's okay—I will try to break it down for you. For me personally, I am a "doer" and a "fixer." If someone asks me for my help, I will agree to help, and in the process, I will do everything in my power to fix whatever the issue was to begin with. I had been investing so much of my time into helping others that I wasn't aware what it was doing to me as an individual. I always help everyone else, even if that means I have to sacrifice my own hopes and dreams. I'm not at all saying helping others is wrong or that you shouldn't do it because you might experience some setbacks personally, but what I do know to be true is that helping others is much more powerful when you can balance helping others as well as helping yourself. Health is not entirely about the amount of fitness you do every day; it is more than that, my friend, and the sooner you narrow down hobbies that make you happy and discover your "why" in life, the sooner you too will be on a path designed to produce positive changes in your own health.

I have been asked how the music you listen to or the people you choose to associate with help you be strong in your health. Have you ever heard the saying, "You are what you eat"? Along the same lines, you also become what you choose to consume or associate with, and that goes for music and the people you choose to do life with. Don't get me wrong, I love me some good old rap music—Tupac, Notorious B.I.G., Nelly, and some old-school Salt-N-Pepa—but playing these songs when I have my five-year-old in the car is not always a good idea; also, playing these songs too much in the car has me thinking I am badass! Seriously, laugh at me now, but some of these artists make me feel invincible, and after listening to some of their songs, I'm up to fight the world as long as I have these songs playing in the background.

The same concept goes for the people I choose to spend my time with. I know now, after experiencing some hard life lessons, that not all people who walk into my life are meant to stay in my life for long periods of time. Sometimes, people are put into your life for a season and maybe not necessarily because you needed them, but because they needed you. When I associate with people who do not encourage me to continue to reach for the stars or who do not understand my "why" to work hard and strive for a better life, I accept that they have opinions, but that does not mean I have to agree with them or put my dreams on hold just because they think I am developing too quickly.

In order for me to have my Cinderella story, I am willing to do whatever it takes: working hard, staying up late to write, working all the overtime to no longer be a slave to debt, staying motivated, and wanting more for my life and my family. I have also learned I need to surround myself with more like-minded people—people who not

Ch. 6 She is *Strong* in her health...

only push their limits and step outside their comfort zones, but who can also encourage me in pushing my limits and stepping out of my comfort zone as well. Just like you can't learn about fitness from someone who is not fit, you can't learn how to grow when you're surrounded by people who are not willing to grow themselves. I am not at all saying you need to drop all your old friends and find new ones, but you do need to stay vigilant in what you share with others who do not share your same values or same goals. Misery loves company, and it's so easy—at least for me—to get all caught up in someone else's problem, and before I know it, now their problem is my problem.

Being strong in my health is not at all something I have mastered. I have so many areas where I can still grow and develop, but learning how to task myself so I can do "all the things" has been essential for me to check things off my to-do lists and bucket list. Being strong in my health is vital if I want to be around when my son and niece have kids of their own. As Dave Ramsey says, "If you will live like no one else, later you can live like no one else." I know this quote was meant for financial purposes, but how convenient is it that this quote can also be used universally when thinking about your own health?

CHAPTER 7
She is *Strong* for her friends . . .

I have not always been a best friend to others. I went through what most young girls probably do in middle school—I picked my friends not because they were supportive and I could tell my deepest, darkest secrets to them, but because they were popular and pretty, and some were great at getting me to live life on the edge. As I write this, I know it sounds awful, and I don't want to say I was ever part of the "mean girls clan," but to some degree, I really may have been. I struggled to fit in, not only with the neighborhood girls, but also with the girls in my middle school. I wanted to be popular, wearing the same clothes they did, styling my hair the same way they did, and even buying the same lotion my friends had. I know—sounds extreme, right?

It wasn't until my first real relationship in eighth grade that the idea of consistently needing to fit in with the so-called cool girls finally subsided. Now, all my energy was wrapped up in my new boyfriend. I had already been living one extreme in how I dealt with the girls, and now I was wrapped up in another extreme in how I handled my first "real" relationship. I made myself available to this boy more than I would like to admit. If he wanted to hang out, I was available. If he wanted to hurt my feelings, it would happen. Looking back, I see that he ran our relationship because I let him, and we were young. As we got into high school, he would almost take it as a threat if I had other friends besides the ones who were closest to our relationship. I would quickly drop friends just so I could hang out with my boyfriend when he'd call. I resented other girls in my high school who even said they thought my boyfriend looked cute. I mean, come on girls, he was *my* boyfriend—*my* property, or so I thought. High school relationships and drama are funny things to look back on, especially because I was sure I was living an adult life in those years.

I know there is no manual for parenting, especially when it comes to parenting your teenage daughter and teaching her right from wrong in relationships, but my friendship with my mother was tested in my early high school days. My parents were okay with the idea of me having a boyfriend at a young age. I'm sure they thought that this too would blow over—I would experience my first heartbreak, and the boy would be history. Oh man, how I wish that had happened, but instead, my boyfriend from eighth grade became serious, and I was sure I would be spending the rest of my life with him. We would say all the things that adults say to one another, talking about how much we loved each other. We would do homework together—literally every waking moment, we would be together, because he was my best friend at the time, next to my mom, of course.

One night, during a heavy make-out session, our kissing led to us doing more adult things—things God doesn't condone before marriage, and I know now our parents wouldn't have condoned it either. But we were in love and just not thinking about any consequences of our actions in that moment. I would give this boy my innocence and my heart, and not just that one time but many times afterward. Honestly, I do not remember specifics, even to this day, of whether we used the pull-out method or condoms or both. What

Ch. 7 She is *Strong* for her friends...

I do remember is I was a teenage girl, and after becoming sexually active with a boy I thought loved me—I mean truly loved me—I became pregnant.

I don't want to dismiss the feelings that in most cases, learning you are pregnant would be an amazing thing and a joyful moment, but as a teenager who'd been told not to be sexually active, I was terrified. I had a job, a serious boyfriend, a car, and responsibilities. But, in reality, I was still just a kid—no way, no how, would I be able to take care of myself and a child. Yes, reader, I hear you loud and clear; I should have thought about that before becoming sexually active. I went through all sorts of stages people in denial go through. I kept thinking the test had to be wrong. I kept thinking my parents were going to kill me. I sucked at keeping secrets, and I'd seen other girls at my school with growing, pregnant bellies, and I was so scared to be one of them. No way would I be one of them, I thought, but truth be told, they were the brave ones. They would learn to blow off the stares and the glares from students and teachers. They were the ones making the true sacrifices in life.

The evening came when I had to tell my mom what I'd done; there were a lot of tears, anger, guilt, and blame. I was sure I was going to hell for what I'd let myself do. I was so scared, and my mom was also so scared for me because she knew what it felt like to be a teen mom. We didn't sit on the idea of me being pregnant for long and definitely did not tell anybody my news. My boyfriend agreed terminating the pregnancy was the best solution for both of us, because heck, what had we been thinking? We were still kids ourselves, and the reality of us being together forever was not realistic.

I can't tell you how many days passed between finding out my pregnancy news and when the nightmare was over, but I do remember feeling overwhelmed and relieved. I remember thinking, "Okay, now things can go back to the way they were before." (Oh, young soul.) Truth be told, nothing would go back to the way it was before. For many years, I would feel like a sinner in my mom's eyes. She never again saw me as her "pure" daughter. My boyfriend no longer seemed to show interest in me like he used to and would lash out by making me jealous with the other girls at school.

Your past does not define you . . .

For years, I faced depression about what had happened and what I had done, and I coped with my thoughts and feelings alone. I wore my smile well. I was sure no one else ever sinned or made mistakes as bad as mine. If no one ever talked about it, then heck, it was almost as if it didn't happen. Knowing what I know now, I shouldn't have let love get in the way of being exactly what I was—just a kid. Knowing what I know now, I am not the person who can make rational decisions based solely on my feelings and have the outcomes turn out well. I will forever have to live with the mistakes I have made, but I can also learn from them. Terminating my pregnancy is not a decision I take lightly, even as an adult; it was a decision I made back in my teenage days that caused me heartache even when it came time to share my pregnancy news years later, when I became pregnant with Urijah. I didn't allow myself to get overly excited, nor did I feel worthy or capable of being chosen to be his mama. I'm being brave in telling such a personal conviction, because it has been on my heart to truly repent for so many years.

After much research, prayers, and scripture readings about my experience, I know God knows my heart better than I ever will. I know he has forgiven all my sins. 1 John 1:9 says, "If we confess our sins, he is faithful and just and will forgive us our sins and purify us from all unrighteousness." For so many years, I allowed myself to be isolated from having any real friendships because I felt unworthy, and I am here writing today, speaking out about a topic that is so frowned upon. If you are reading this and experiencing these feelings in real time, I want you to know you are not alone, and your life is not over. You have options even in your darkest hour, when you feel like there are none. It is okay to forgive yourself and ask for grace when it comes to some of the decisions you have made in your life. You, my friend, are strong just to ask for help in your journey to heal from such trauma; I truly believe that.

It wouldn't be till the end of my junior year that I would try very hard to take a break from being in a serious relationship. During this time, I focused my attention on extra activities at the school, such as cheerleading, tennis, and the swim team, just so I could make new friends. Being involved in these extra activities helped me develop real relationships with other girls my age.

It wasn't until I fully let go of all the relationship drama and all the jealousy that I finally started to enjoy my years in high school. I finally started developing relationships with all types of people at my school. I didn't care anymore about my social status—if I fit in or if I didn't. I was just proud of myself for finally being okay in my own skin and not having to live up to the expectations of the other girls, boys, or adults that were in my life at the time.

True friendships were made in my last two years of high school, and while I am not proud of how I treated some of my best friends back in high school, their love for me was evident then and even more evident now. They have shown me time and time again what it means to be strong as a true friend. These ladies are the first to tell me my faults. These ladies are the first people to cheer me on when I am tackling a new journey. These ladies are the ones I can laugh with, cry with, and pray with when life gets overwhelming. This group of ladies has seen me fail and hit rock bottom, and they are also a part of my journey now. I love you ladies so much for showing me true friendship, even when I wasn't the best of friend back to you. There is strength in having healthy friendships, women helping women, and having each other's backs when times get tough.

True friends are hard to find…

While I am lucky enough to have my childhood friends, I am also equally as lucky to have friendships that have developed in my church life. Some of these are newer friendships, meaning I have been in their lives less than a year, but some of my church friendships have also led into some of the best mentoring I have ever experienced in my adult life. When I started my faith journey five years ago, the head of the children's ministry was one of the first people I met at North Metro, partly because I had a one-year-old and a three-year-old going with me every Sunday, and I wanted to be sure the classes they would be in were safe and that the staff knew me by name. (Yes, you're thinking correctly—I am that helicopter mom.) I also wanted to know the head of the children's ministry, because I was very much interested in serving in this area of the church. I will be forever grateful to Sunny, as she met me in some of my darkest and most confusing times in my adult life. She gently guided me, always with God's word. She made herself available for coffee or a girls' night out when I needed a friend the most. I watched Sunny build trust with the families who dropped off their babies every Sunday; family by family, Sunny knew the moms, dads, and kids by name, and she always had a smile on her face. Short-staffed and all, she remained positive with the words, "God will provide," and he did always come through for her.

When Sunny left the children's ministry position, it was evident parents weren't so trusting anymore in dropping off their smaller babies. I was a volunteer in the program, and I got to witness the decline, and it broke my heart. I wasn't sure how to fix the problem, and quite honestly, my own family was in a season where we were having to make a decision—did we stay at North Metro or move to a church closer to home, one that offered services on days other than just Sundays? My family and I moved churches, and it wasn't until recently that I fit all the puzzle pieces together and realized just how important it is, to have the right people serving in the right places in the church.

Ch. 7 She is *Strong* for her friends...

Sunny taught me strength in being compassionate and caring with our church families; she showed me what it meant to be in community with our church and that volunteers truly resemble the heart and soul of the church. I don't reach out to Sunny as much as I should, but her friendship has left an imprint on my heart.

Other friendships that have blossomed from church are with people I have met while volunteering. Hearing all their personal testimonies and what led them to the church always inspires me. I only get to catch up with some of these friends once a month, when we serve together, but it's always reassuring to see a familiar face when I walk into the church. Recently in my faith journey, my husband and I became open to the idea of joining a small group, but neither one of us had been a part of any type of support group as an adult. I, being the social butterfly in our relationship, only had to think on this for maybe a day or so, but it wasn't until the first meeting, where my husband experienced it for himself, that he completely felt like this small group would be okay for us to continue going to.

If you have never participated in a small group and are reading this, I encourage you to find a small group in your community. It does not have to be faith based—it can be a support group that helps you battle addiction, it can be a support group to help you with a long-term or short-term medical condition—but the moment you find like-minded people who are experiencing what you are and can support you in your struggles and celebrate with you when you overcome a hurdle, life as you know it changes. The world, for once, does not seem so harsh. Your perception of the people you share life with changes. You will no longer feel isolated and alone!

Shawn and I have found this to be true while attending our marrieds' Bible study group. I went into the group thinking two extremes could be true: One, we would be met with other couples who had their entire lives put neatly together, seeing no flaws in themselves and looking to judge or create division within the group right away.

Or we would be met with opens arms and accepted exactly the way we were, with no judgments about the way we parent or how much money we have. Now I admit, those were two extreme thoughts I had going into our first small group session, but my thoughts were exactly what I said—just thoughts. Turns out, in this season of our lives, we needed this group, we needed their positivity, we needed their prayers, and we were overall grateful for their friendship and support they provided in a way our other friends or family members could not provide at this time of our lives. I am fully confident there is no coincidence in the timing of when we joined our marrieds' Bible study. Our friendship with this group is still so fresh and new; I've found strength in telling my story to complete strangers. Life is hard and is meant to be shared in community with others, and I truly believe 100 percent that God used this group to soften not only my heart but my husband's stubborn heart too.

Practice consistency . . .

Good ole social media, am I right? I didn't realize the power of social media until I started blogging. I would advertise my blog on my local Facebook moms' group pages, Bible study group pages, and my own personal page, and what do you know, my writings and my content took off. Soon, I had more Facebook friend requests than I knew what to do with. I try really hard not to overflow my page with personal pictures of the kids, but as we do have lots of family all over the States, posting pictures of the kids every now and then helps family to see that our kids are no longer babies.

Accepting complete strangers prompted mama bear to really think about how I could support my readers who truly do want to get to know more about me and the stories behind my daily blogs. While I realize not everyone on social media is who they say they are, this is an ongoing battle, and eventually I will not be able to screen everyone who sends me a friend request. It's also true that we will have an entire upcoming generation of children who never

Ch. 7 She is *Strong* for her friends...

asked for their pictures to be put on the internet to begin with. When they start middle school or high school, even though they may not have personally put naked baby photos of themselves on the internet—maybe their mom or grandma did—that in itself can and may be used as blackmail.

By educating moms, dads, and caregivers on the dangers that social media presents, we will all be better equipped in making conscious decisions as to which pictures we choose to share of our children, knowing just how far that one photo can really go. I follow other successful writers on social media, and it does not appear to me this is a subject most writers or successful people in general have a handle on themselves. It is one thing to want to protect your children, but protecting your children too much and not allowing them to fail or get their feelings hurt sometimes will only hurt them when they become adults and eventually they have to live life without you, the parent always protecting them.

I am choosing to write about my social media friends because we live in a day and age where the idea is that to be fully successful and reach people by the masses, you need to do Facebook Live videos, post to all social media outlets (Twitter, Snapchat, Instagram, etc.) and create YouTube content. People (me included) will spend their time with like-minded people who share a common agenda—a common value system. Your values are what make people want to work with you and only you. Honestly, it takes time to build a true social media platform, and building a platform well means establishing from the get-go the type of culture you are looking to build. If your message is to spread inspiration and encouragement, followers (I do hate using that word) will be scanning your personal social media outlets for everything you say that you're about, and the minute they find something that does not fit the mold you claim to be, the trust of that particular social media follower is broken. Gone are the days of getting on TV or getting published in a magazine (I mean, that still happens, but less and less often, I suppose). We as a society are so busy these days that audiobooks are replacing books and Netflix is replacing cable TV. I write about my social media friends because although they may not be intertwined with my daily life hour by hour, they choose to spend some of their time learning about me, reading my blogs, and following my content. Learning to be strong for my friends on social media has been just as important as learning how to be strong for the friends who may need me physically.

Time is something we don't get back; once it's gone, it's gone. I recognize the people who take the time to find me on Facebook and like a post or like a blog—heck, when they share my content on their own social media pages, I want to acknowledge that I see it and I appreciate it so much. If there is anything you take away from this chapter, know and understand that friendship comes in so many forms. It's our mindset that limits us in how we define friendship. I find the mindset topic to be intriguing in itself, but when we are willing to expand, grow, and accept a new mindset, the sky's the limit.

Who you do life with matters...

The word *friend* most of the time references people whom you have grown up with and maybe people you interact with daily or on a monthly basis. But the word *friend* is also defined as companionship, closeness, understanding, and fellowship. Who else better fits all these definitions than my husband, Shawn. Now, if you are not at all prepared to hear why this man I do life with is so freaking amazing, I give you full permission to skip this section, because, you guys, it's going to get mushy. I want to write about the friendship Shawn and I truly do share with one another, and I want to finally give this man the praise he deserves to hear (okay, read) from me. This man stepped into some big shoes the night he met me at our local bar. I know I poured out my entire life story in a matter of a few hours (sorry, not sorry). Most men would have found all that information overwhelming and left the evening wondering

Ch. 7 She is *Strong* for her friends...

what the heck had just happened, but Shawn didn't do that to me. Instead, Shawn built trust with me, helping not only me but also my entire family move into a new home. He continued to build that trust when he stayed by my side while I went through bankruptcy court and lost every material thing I have ever owned. We have the relationship we have because we were friends first. Even after we made the decision to become "official," Shawn has never held me back from my dreams, even my expensive ones (*cough*, my college degree). He has always believed in me, even during the many times when I could not believe in myself. His common sense and guidance in life are things I try daily to not take for granted. Till the day I die, he will be my life companion, as we complement each other well. He can straight up tell me the hard truths and the things that need to change, but he can also be the best listener and a shoulder to cry on when I need him most.

While there have been many seasons where Shawn and I seem inseparable, the two of us work because we can acknowledge each one of us has different likes and wants than the other. We are completely okay with spending countless hours together and are also comfortable spending much-needed time apart. As a couple, we see the importance of not only having mutual couple friends but also having our individual friendships as well. I can't expect my husband to be able to fulfill all my wants and desires for the rest of my life, and vice versa. Our relationship thrives because it has never been based off of jealously, even in our dating days. I have seen women show interest in him, and he has seen guys show interest in me. Our relationship also thrives because the two of us constantly work on ways we can better communicate with one another. I may be beating a dead horse, but, you guys, communication in any relationship or friendship is important, and knowing where you lack personally when it comes to communicating effectively can help you immensely.

Shawn has been our family's primary provider for many years, and since he's in HVAC, where people need him at all different times of the year, I have witnessed him solving heater and AC problems over the phone. Also, going to work functions and hearing customers rave about Shawn and getting a chance to see him through someone else's eyes has been powerful in itself. I can appreciate Shawn for who he is. We also work because we are not in the business of trying to change one another. So many people we meet and have interacted with have all these gripes about why their spouse needs to change this or change that. But the honest truth is that change will happen in the relationship when you learn to focus all that change not on your spouse but on *yourself*. What I have realized after so much personal development on myself is that the people around me started to take notice, and some were even curious about the books I was reading, the podcasts I was listening to, and so forth. Once my husband realized as well that this was not just a phase—that I was all in—he has learned in his own way and understood that there is a better and more fulfilling way to live.

    I learned from my mom and dad the type of relationship I wanted to have with my spouse. I also learned from my parents the parts of a relationship I didn't want to have. Personally learning from past relationships with other people, I've reflected back on the times we worked well together and what I would change regarding why we failed. I used to be the jealous girlfriend back in high school. I used to be the person who would only have you as a friend if you could help my social status. Living life this way could never fulfill me. It could never lead me to successfully figuring out my "why" in life. I learned strength in really learning and understanding what it takes to be strong as a friend and companion. The grass is not always greener on the other side; the grass is greener where you water it!

CHAPTER 8
She is *Strong* for herself...

I woke up on time to get ready for the day. I left the house on time so I could get to work. Then—bam!—wouldn't you know it? Traffic galore! I had been on time, and now I would be late for work.

That morning, I had to giggle at myself because I knew the moment I saw traffic, my old self would have let that sight ruin my day or at least my morning. My old self would have not been able to brush off the minor traffic jam.

This leads me to talk about why your past does not define you. It is really nice when other people remind you that "you, my friend, are loved." Whether I am winning or whether I am failing miserably, I have people in my circle who love me and tell me so daily. I usually don't hop on every good idea I have, partly because my old self was afraid of failure and partly because I am not a sales person, and most of my so-called good ideas involve some sort of sales scheme. But last night, I came to the realization that I don't pursue good ideas because, quite frankly, it's hard to put myself out there. Truly exposing yourself to the community you live in, work in, and play in has high stakes, and for me, if I fail, then part of me feels like

I am failing my entire community. I do realize this idea may be rash, and I can't put the world on my shoulders like that. But this realization made me see that I no longer put myself in a position where I might risk failing my community. I no longer put myself in that place where I assume I am going to fail. I don't resonate with that person anymore. Failing at something does not make you a failure; it leads you to try new things, and that, my friend, is brave.

Thinking back on my life and the countless ways I've failed is not fun for me, but the amount of knowledge that came from those experiences will stay with me my entire life. I learned in my early twenties I didn't fit the mold of the so-called norm that surrounded me. My early twenties showed me a lot of heartache, worry, and guilt for not meeting the standards and goals that some of my close friends were meeting. Looking back now, I compared myself *way* too much: Why was I not happily married? Why was I not having babies? Why was I not succeeding in college? Dang it, why was I not enjoying epic nights out?

My reality was that I was overweight, unhappily married, and consumed with stuff I couldn't afford, and the way this ended for me was in divorce and bankruptcy by the time I was twenty-two. In this season of my life, I wasn't living. I didn't see the bigger picture. I had no faith and no hope in my future, but when I failed, I sure failed. The only constant in my life at that time was my job, and man, was I good at my job. But shortly after my epic life fail, my job fell apart too. I was fired. I argued, "You can't fire me! I am one of your top producers! I already have my dress for the Christmas party. I've invested so much time into your company."

Well, my friend, none of my good deeds saved my job that day—none of my good deeds for that company saved my pride that day either. At this time in my life, I didn't have children, although I was in a newfound relationship with my now husband, Shawn. He knew just as well as I did that I was not happy. It took a lot of work for me to get out of my funk.

Ch. 8 She is *Strong* for herself...

Looking back at my time of chaos, I see that being let go from a job I had put so much of my own identity into was a blessing; this was a moment when God showed up for me, and I'd had no idea. I ended up losing my job in November that year. I learned to pick myself up and to quit feeling sorry for myself and my situation. The moment I picked myself up from the pits, I found out I was pregnant, and that, folks, is where my journey all started. You, my friend, are not defined by your past, by your failures, by your career, or by what others think of you. You don't have to live under the weight of comparing yourself or your situation to anyone else. My prayer today is that you would practice forgiveness—forgiving yourself for your past and forgiving others for what they did to you in your past. Doing this will help you not only let go of all that negative energy but also allow you to focus on what your future holds for you. Practice what it means to truly live and be thankful in the Lord and all his gifts. You got this!

My story is not at all simple, and the many people who know me personally know I wear multiple hats, and I mean multiple hats all in a day's work. I am a mama, a wife, a daughter, a sister, an aunt, a coworker, and a sister in Christ, just to name a few, and while I strive daily to wear all my hats well, there are days when I choose to pick maybe two or three hats and do those duties really well, and I tend to not worry about the rest. Usually when this happens, and I am choosing my hats for the day, it's because it's payday. Some people may be reading this and say, "Girl, your answer is a budget! Make yourself a monthly budget." Oh, honey, I so do this! I am the one who uses Microsoft Excel and will balance my funds out to the last penny. What I'm getting at is that for me, regardless of whether we are in a great season or a really crappy season, the topic of money creates a feeling of uncertainty in me that I do not like. I do not like payday because it forces me to think about this uncertainty—triggers me, if you will. There is probably some underlying psychological trauma explaining why I feel this way about money, as it has always been a subject I have been naive about for as far back as I can remember. But it's also a subject I continually work to be educated on. Heck, I even got my bachelor's degree in business administration with an emphasis in accounting. Can anyone relate to this feeling?

This leads me to talk about accepting your life's uncertainties. Whatever your life's uncertainties are, know it is completely okay and healthy to not know all the answers. It is completely healthy to let life take you "by the balls" as you wing it. In my own life, I have come to see that the more I plan, the more my plans fall apart. My obsessive self wants to believe I am in control, when in reality, I am not at all in control. As I have said before, God's in control, and he knows my needs even before I realize what they are. It's up to me to remain obedient and truly accept my life's uncertainties, whatever they may be.

Are you still with me, friend? Have you ever thought about what your life's destiny will be? That everything you have been through in your life—good and bad, planned and unplanned—will all lead up to one moment in life when you realize you're exactly where you need to be, because this was all part of his bigger plan? I participated in an online Bible study (shout-out to all my *Beautifully Brave* ladies!), and if you are having a hard time resonating with me and my thoughts, I encourage you to go pick up Beth Moore's *Esther* Bible series (and no, I get no kickback from saying her name or the name of her Bible series). There is a workbook along with videos you can purchase, and I encourage you to learn more about Esther and her story. The Esther story is empowering for so many reasons; in the Bible, it brings to light that women are placed on this earth for a bigger purpose. In the story of Esther, the way she handled herself and her personal trials saved an entire Jewish community. Trust me when I tell you, I hadn't picked up a Bible in my adult life before this series started, and friend, I can't describe the clarity, the freedom, and the peace her story will bring to your own life and how you feel about your life's uncertainties.

Ch. 8 She is *Strong* for herself...

I realize I am asking a lot, and I also know that accepting life's uncertainties may be a daily struggle for many of us. It will take a lot of conscious effort in the beginning to learn to just accept your life's uncertainties, but that's okay. Be kind to yourself! That is what personal development is all about.

Have you ever felt like you were chasing after your dreams instead of living out your dreams? I have! My husband, one of the hardest-working men I know, quit his job of seven years back in June. It was not at all an easy decision, as he has been the primary provider for our family for our entire relationship. But I was no longer willing to risk my husband's health for a job he no longer felt satisfied with. My husband is a very smart man, and a handy man at that! I knew he would bounce back from unemployment quickly, but so far, we are five months in. He has been applying and given hope for new beginnings, and then something will come up, and he's given excuses for why he has not ended up being hired or getting the job. So here we sit, patiently waiting, thinking we took one step forward and now are taking ten steps backward and starting at square one.

During this season of unemployment, my husband and I agreed to start a Financial Peace class through our local church. (It really is a Dave Ramsey financial boot camp.) I have to admit, I was so nervous to even sign us up, because in reality, am I really ready to take on dealing with all our debt at a time like this? We are currently living off of one income—do I dare take on something I am not 100 percent convinced I can follow through on? Well, we signed up. We signed up for a nine-week Dave Ramsey financial boot camp, and watching the first video was not so bad. I actually had not realized Dave Ramsey was so faith based. Our homework assignment and baby step one was to save up a thousand dollars and put it away. Part two was to complete the Quick-Start Budget form, write down an assessment of our total nonmortgage debt and the amount of total liquid assets we had available, and, lastly, write down how many open credit card accounts we had.

I have mentioned this before in blog posts, but my relationship with money is not at all healthy. I dread paying bills, but I will do it. I take on the stress of paying bills not only for my household but also for my parents, so that stress is multiplied. You can imagine my concern just trying to tackle this first homework assignment. I was a huge ball of anxiety, and when I get like that, ladies and gents, all I want to do is eat! Not just healthy food, but comfort food. I have worked on myself enough to know money is one of my triggers, though. I won't give in anymore and eat away my worries, but days like this definitely make it very hard to get through, and I am exhausted by the time eight o'clock comes around.

Some would say, "But wait, you signed up for this willingly!" Yes, I did, and you want to know why? Because I like the feeling I get when I give all my worries up to the Lord, and giving up my finances is no exception. I want to feel the type of freedom that comes from truly giving my finances up to the Lord. I have never been taught how to manage my money well or how to lean into my faith when things are hard; instead, I treat money as if I am in control. We have good credit, so many would think I am indeed in control, but it's not always so straightforward. Yes, I can pay bills and temporarily save, but I no longer want—and my family no longer wants—to just get by, and I don't have the tools to make such a big goal happen for myself or for my family. So I signed us up for financial boot camp!

I do plan to trust the Dave Ramsey process, but I also can't shake the feeling I am taking some steps backward in retraining my brain to learn all about money and saving. If I am being honest, this part of personal development is not fun right now. I'm sorry if I sound like such a sap! But these are my thoughts, and I have been aching to get them out of my head and onto paper.

I am also reading *Odd(ly) Enough* by my girl, Carolanne Miljavac, and tonight, while reading chapter five, it hit me; all these thoughts I am having about taking one step forward and ten steps back—this is indeed what the enemy sounds like. The enemy is good at making us feel like we are not enough or not qualified or that what we are doing is not enough.

I fully support my husband in this journey of unemployment. Do I think the jobs he has interviewed for that sounded promising were at all a waste of time? No, I don't, and actually, this last potential job has in some ways changed the way we "share our faith" together. This season of unemployment has made us communicate better and open our hearts to love a new church and for our family to follow Christ every day and not just on Sunday.

The enemy also knows the fears I have when it comes to money, as I already have *married*, *divorced* and *bankrupt* stamped on my forehead. As I am making strides to changing the future of my family tree, I want to retrain my ways of thinking regarding money so I am better equipped to teach my son and my niece how to succeed when they are older. The enemy wants me to give in and beat myself up about all the ways I am not living perfectly. I am writing this out on paper to fight back those thoughts. To fight back the negative self-talk.

I know I am not alone in my way of thinking, and I hope my words will inspire others to fight back and not give up as well! We were not given this life to constantly feel defeated! We will persevere; God's way always wins! Please know you're not alone in this fight, and you're not alone in your thoughts. I still see God showing up for me and my family with the doors he is keeping closed and the new doors he is allowing to open. He is showing me I am more than capable of writing a book, writing on my blog, and preparing my body, heart, and soul for hard work so I can live in complete freedom, not only in his word, but in financial freedom as well. But it won't be handed to me. It will take hard work, consistency, and patience like I've never known to fully trust and believe that God can do all things.

Facebook Memories was quick to remind me I haven't always been so grateful. I haven't always been living out the best version of myself. It took courage to finally wake up and step out of my comfort zone, which has led to the writing of this book. Looking back, I see that my old self was so naive! I know I say that word a lot, but seriously, I was!

I remember being a senior in high school and thinking I had the world at my fingertips. I was going to graduate high school, go to college, finish my degree in four years, find an amazing husband, get our house with the white picket fence, have lots of babies (that I could afford), find one job that I would turn into my career, do it well, and then have an amazing retirement when I was seventy. That was going to be my life! That was going to be my happy ending!

Reality check: that is not at all where my life was heading. When I was a senior in high school, my home life was falling apart. My mom was fighting breast cancer, she was having multiple surgeries that would save her life, and my parents were going through a nasty separation that led to a divorce. My brother was going through an identity crisis (he desperately longed to know who he was and where he came from), and I was accepted to CU Boulder here in Colorado, where I'd live in the dorms on scholarships and student loans. My boyfriend at the time was *scary*, to say the least. My life was not at all going how I'd pictured it. My freshman year of college didn't get any better. Ask my mom; I was impossible to wake up on time in high school (my old self hated mornings), and once I was in college with no parental control, I struggled every day to get up for class. I quickly learned my professors didn't care if I showed up to class—then why should I care? I barely endured my first year as a college student. I received a few Fs in that time as well. But stepping out of my comfort zone just was not an option for me. I was doing the day-to-day routine that I thought every college student did at that time. I lived this way a long time, and not happily. But I followed this trend through my twenties.

Ch. 8 She is *Strong* for herself...

Fast-forward to six years ago, when I was a new mom. My niece had officially been adopted into our family. An identity crisis hit me like nothing I had ever experienced before.

Fast-forward to a year ago. I was asked to be in a wedding—my dear friend's wedding. A girl I had known since grade school. She sent me a cute package in the mail, asking me to be her bridesmaid. I had never been a bridesmaid before, and I was in no shape to go try on bridesmaid dresses. Remember, I was the girl who had struggled with weight ever since I graduated high school. But with that reasoning alone, I could not tell her no. I truly wanted to be in her wedding, and I was going to do whatever it took to look good in whatever dress she wanted me in. In August of 2017, I stepped out of my comfort zone and joined a gym called HIITBox. I talked to my trainer and told him my goals and my fears, and he and the HIITBox trainers worked my butt off. Besides giving birth, I have never felt like I wanted to die, but when I was in their classes—oh girl, bring it!

I have been doing so much self-work. What that looks like for me is attending and participating in personal development conferences a few times a year. I have signed up for life coaching, discussing hard life topics such as accepting your past, perspectives, and creating a road map of how I will achieve my dreams. I have also done self-work when it comes to how I handle finances and setting boundaries with friends and family. I couldn't hide all this self-work if I tried. I encourage you to really look into things that get you out of your comfort zone. We grow the most when we're not comfortable with our surroundings; we grow the most when we laugh at ourselves, even just a little bit. Put yourself in uncomfortable situations; do things you thought you would never do because you didn't think you fit the mold. By doing this, you show yourself just how truly brave you can be, and you, my reader, have it in you to be brave, be strong, and do great things!

So many distractions . . .

I used to journal a lot in middle school and into high school, and somewhere I lost my way. I remember I tried to pick it back up once I became pregnant in 2012—that lasted about six months before I let life distractions get in the way. Think for a second about the people in your life who show confidence, who speak words of wisdom, and who bring you overwhelming peace when they talk to you, and, for whatever reason, you can't quite put your finger on why they make you feel this way. I'll tell you why: because confidence, my friend, is beautiful!

Confidence can make a person glow from the inside out. Truly confident people don't necessarily have all the answers you're looking for; instead, they have the ears to listen to your sorrows or your outbursts of joy, and they have a heart to give, even if they have nothing but their time to give you. My pastor refers to these ideas as the fruit of the Holy Spirit. In case you are not familiar with the fruit of the Spirit, here you go: love, joy, peace, patience, kindness, goodness, faithfulness, gentleness, and consistency (self-control). Nowhere in here do you see beauty, body figure, or size—do you see where I am going with this? The fruit of the Spirit helps a person find their true inner confidence, and that, you guys, is beautiful.

I follow quite a few ladies on social media, and every day they inspire me and teach me new things. Sometimes, while I am watching their videos or listening to their podcasts, I think to myself, "Man, she is speaking directly to me."

Recently I have been listening to Rachel Hollis, and I love her idea of the power of self-talk. Self-talk can truly be a very powerful tool when used correctly and practiced a lot. Practicing self-talk is a task in itself—at first I felt funny and kind of stupid, and I was not feeling like I was inspiring myself at all. I actually thought this might lead me to set up a psych visit for myself! But the more I practiced this self-talk, the more things in my life changed; I started blogging

Ch. 8 She is *Strong* for herself...

to the world, and my attitude changed in how I treat myself and how I let others treat me. Even the most important items on my to-do list, which I have prayed would change, are changing.

I have said from day one that you, my friend, have the power to change. You, my friend, have the power to change the course of how your life is going. You, my friend, have the world at your fingertips if you allow your willingness to change take complete control over your spirit.

This has been a true experience of freedom and peace like I have never experienced before. I encourage you to take the time to find a podcast, find someone on social media who inspires you, find a personal development article, and just start reading or watching. Listen to their wisdom; listen to their testimonies. Write down what similarities you and the people you've chosen have in common. My friend, you have it within you to be confident and beautiful. Take that first step!

I am honestly not sure if the people who read my writing are mostly women or men. But it doesn't matter, because my writing can be read and understood no matter your gender, background, beliefs, etc. I truly do feel like diversity with my readers is important. Today, I've had consistency on my heart. I have thought about this concept not only with my blog but also in writing this book. Narrowing down my daily activities, each Monday through Friday, it is a given that I'll go to work for eight hours a day. Why? Because I need to make money, and my job allows me to do just that. But within that eight-hour day, I get to choose to work hard and show up for my coworkers, who need not only my physical body but my spunk, the right attitude, and a positive mindset to make our day together go as smoothly as possible. The families I serve also need my energy, my spunk, and my wisdom to help them figure out which insurance program would best fit the needs of their families. I really don't have time to waste on my "off" days. I can clearly remember one weekend where I was on fire—serving in my community, cleaning the entire house, and revamping my blog—and then leave it to Netflix to distract me. It's not every weekend my husband and I get time to just sit and start a Netflix series, but while I was doing "all the things," my husband would be flipping through Netflix, trying to find a good show to watch. He finally settled on a show called *The Flash*. We got sucked into this show so fast! One episode led to ten episodes and even a second season the following day. When Monday rolled around, I could not for the life of me figure out why I felt so sluggish, or why getting back into my normal routine of writing was just not flowing.

During this time, I was also working through the book *High Performance Habits*—so much information just in chapter one. The author, Brendon Burchard, has so many good tips about setting up a daily routine and increasing productivity. He writes about things I would have never thought of when it comes to the way I am wired, the way I do life, and the way I market myself. If you are looking for a game changer for yourself or your business, check out Brendon's weekly podcasts and audiobook. In the audiobook, he talks about taking his HPI (Hogan Personality Inventory) assessment test—I will admit, tests give me anxiety, no matter what type of test it is. I literally freeze or feel like I will answer the questions the wrong way. Taking a *High Performance Habits* test did not sound fun to me, but I buckled down and completed it. It breaks down your scores into six *High Performance Habit* scores: clarity, energy, necessity, productivity, influence, and courage. Can you guess where it showed that I needed improvement? Necessity. My results say, "Low levels of necessity make it hard to turn off Netflix and get stuff done." You guys, I couldn't make this stuff up if I tried. That weekend, I had been on fire, but I'd also spent a full day and a half binge-watching Netflix, and then I'd had a hard time regaining my focus on my goals.

What I am getting at, my friend, is that consistency is key. I am not wired to have one "off" day when it comes to goal setting. And while "off" days are inevitable, those days—however many

Ch. 8 She is *Strong* for herself...

I may have in a month—may lead to setbacks with the ultimate goals I have set for myself. Today and every day from here on out, I will practice consistency and remember just how important it is for my personal development. I encourage you, friend, to take the time to learn more about yourself. Take the time to truly find what makes you tick. I know I sound like a broken record, but the breakthroughs you will discover about yourself will help you reach your goals faster and, in turn, have you living out the best version of you.

The ripple effect . . .

Having the right mindset can be such a powerful tool. Even on the days when I am not convinced the day will go my way, or when I can feel Satan knocking on my door, I take a deep breath, meditate, and really focus on changing my mindset. Sometimes this exercise only has to happen a few times throughout the day; other days, refocusing on my mindset needs to happen every hour for my sanity. What I am seeing in myself is change like nothing I have ever experienced. We have all heard the saying "practice what you preach," right? Those things that we preach about usually take the *most* practice. I warned you before, I listen to a lot of Rachel Hollis right now, but honestly guys, her words are gold—true wisdom I need to hear and learn from. Not surprisingly, she said something in her podcast that helped me, and I am sure that talking about it could help out a lot of people who struggle with anxiety and depression.

I listen to various Audible books, podcasts, and radio talks—it is not surprising when something good comes on, and I am alone in my car, to find myself nodding and talking back the speaker who doesn't even know I exist. So many personal-development speakers talk about showing gratitude; when gratitude is shown correctly and developed into a habit, a person finds it difficult to be bothered, worried, or concerned about a subject that may very well have made them mad in the past.

Coming from a family that suffers from mental health issues ranging from trauma, PTSD, depression, and anxiety, I realize the risk for myself and why it is so important for me to know and learn the signs of when to ask for help, which includes listening to my body about when it's appropriate for me to take a time-out or all in all remove myself from a situation. I refuse to allow my mental health to be put into overdrive, as I have watched too many loved ones suffer far too much from not tackling the root of the problem to begin with.

As I move forward in this journey called life, my goal for myself is to live with intentionality and, when doing so, to really put into practice all that I preach. When I say, "Yes, I will pray for you," I want my friends and family to know that I am truly praying for them. When I say, "Be slow to anger," I will remind myself in times of rage or fear why being slow to anger is so important. I want to live my life honorably and truly practice what I preach—in my faith, with my finances, and in my day-to-day tasks.

The reason I write is to inspire and to let it be known that no one, and I mean no one, should struggle with their demons alone. This life we live is hard, and knowing there are people who can tell those hard truths and overcome such hardships gives me hope, not only for my life but humanity in general. I listened to a *RISE Together Podcast* episode that said, "Kids do not listen to what you say; they listen to what you do," and I have seen this idea reflected in how my son learns more from my actions than from what I tell him to do. One night, my husband and I were talking openly about what we fight about the most, which, surprisingly, was how we parent our son. Now, the people who know us personally may think, "Really? But you guys are great parents!" And to them, I would say, "Thank you!"

But there is also a hard truth both my husband and I have realized, which is that we do not at all parent our son the same way. My husband is sure I baby our six-year-old too much, while I am equally sure my husband can be too hard and insensitive to our child's feelings. One thing I've learned early on in our parenting journey is that it is completely okay to not parent the same way, and neither Dad's way nor Mom's way of parenting is right or wrong. My husband may not give our son a bath the way I like it done—my husband may not console our child's tears the way I like it done—but that does not mean the way he does things is wrong. In this way of thinking, though, I am fully aware of just how much our child is watching us as parents—the way we handle arguments, stress, fitness, life's daily tasks—and he is learning by Mom's and Dad's actions and our responses to handling this thing called life.

My response to my husband is that while we may not parent, console, or do things the same way, and that's all okay, we also need to be more vigilant with the fact that little eyes are paying more attention to our actions. This even goes for how we discipline. Have you ever heard of a ripple effect? Usually we hear this used when scientists are talking about water or a science experiment. Recently, I learned this idea could also be applied to parenting, which brings me to my real-life ripple effect. Our son, Urijah, will learn to speak how we speak just by watching the way his dad and I talk to each other every day. He will learn to speak the bad words exactly the ways we use the bad words. Yes, he might not be driving now because he is only six years old, but he is actively watching Mom and Dad wear our seat belts when we are in the car, texting while driving, or just being on the phone in general while driving. Our actions now as parents will ultimately shape the driver he will become later. Trust me, I am aware of all these actions, and I say them not because I have mastered doing all these things correctly; rather, I am saying these things out loud to fellow parents struggling with the parenting topic. You, my friend, are not alone.

Admitting my husband and I have some areas of parenting that need work is not going to cause us to break up; rather, it will encourage us to work even harder to fix our flawed behaviors. The ripple effect not only happens with the things my son sees inside our home but also with the things we do outside of the home—things like small group, workouts, and serving our community, just to name a few. My faith journey as an adult and a mom started a little over five years ago. But it started just like I said—for me. When my son was little, I would bring him and my niece to church services. These last few months, God has been hard at work, changing our family dynamic and really bringing us back to ground zero, to what's important. I say God has done this, because for the last five years, I have prayed for my husband to open up his heart at least to the idea of church, and not just on a holiday. I realized early on I am not powerful enough to change a grown man's heart, nor am I a pushy, nagging wife to force my husband to want exactly the things I want.

One weekend in October, I witnessed all my prayers answered. God had been listening all these years. He was listening and working not only in me but also in my husband. We served at my son's elementary school together for a Halloween function—I worked the craft table, and my husband served food to the community. Then we served together again that Sunday, working at our community's Trunk or Treat event held by a church both of us would later attend together to complete an entire four-week church series. This was a huge deal, as my husband was not at all an avid churchgoer, and I will give God the glory on this one!

Talk about a ripple effect in the making when it comes to our son. How much more powerful is it showing our son the importance of becoming a man of faith, when not only one of his parents lives by God's word, but both his parents are working to be obedient? As his parents, we only want the best life for our son. We want him to work hard for his dreams; we would love for him to be a man of faith, to be a leader in his community. We can tell him we want all these things for him and have it go in one ear and out the other, or we can show him how all these things are possible and educate him on how he can make all this happen for himself as he gets older.

Ch. 8 She is *Strong* for herself...

Do you see just how powerful a ripple effect can be? I sure can, and this gives me reassurance as to why I am working so hard on myself, on my attitude, on my faith, and on my communication with my husband. I have learned to be strong for myself through all my life experiences; although my story is still nowhere close to being finished, I have found a sense of peace by just being able to write and finally get my words out of my head and on paper. Reader, I truly want such a peace for you too.

This season is temporary . . .

If you have read this far into my book, you have read time and time again my frustrations when it comes to money, and for me, that started at quite a young age. While I don't at all want to sound like a broken record, I also want you to truly understand why this subject is so near and dear to my heart. As an adult, I have come to terms with the fact that I have some serious insecurities surrounding money and how I have handled money throughout my life. I truly feel like I lit a spark inside myself by starting Dave Ramsey's Financial Peace boot camp. I have come to the realization I know what it takes to get a good credit score, and when balances start racking up and getting out of hand, I also know the word *refinance* to help consolidate the debt that somehow grew out of control. Let's just call me the refinance queen! Needless to say, since starting this Dave Ramsey journey, I have had to retrain and reteach myself on everything—and I mean everything—I once thought to be true about money. Oh my word, you guys, I am not going to lie to you—it has been one of the hardest things I have ever tackled individually and in my relationship. Because it is such a challenge doing the weekly homework, creating the weekly budget, and holding not only myself but my husband accountable to our financial goals, I sometimes just cry because this journey is so hard. I fully understand why people quit and drop out of the program, because dang it, it is so freaking hard.

Last night, as I was writing to my gym trainer to cancel my HIITBox membership, I was feeling pretty defeated. Let me explain. In August 2017, I went to my trainer, wanting to change my life and wanting to develop better habits. My health was really poor. I was overweight, comfort eating all the time, and rocking the scale as a prediabetic. It was bad! Then I met Adam, a local trainer, and his success rate in our community was amazing. Everyone said the workouts were hard, but they didn't die, and oddly enough the challenge made going fun! It took paying someone else to tell me to do jumping jacks and to push me to run in order for my life to change. I have dropped thirty pounds in the last year.

I found my inner strength to become healthy physically and emotionally and to stay healthy for no one else but myself. HIITBox was the push I needed to make life changes, so having to even temporarily cancel such a key contributor to what I have accomplished in this last year hurt my heart and soul to my core. Even writing these words now makes me fight back tears. Adam, being the amazing trainer he is, wrote something last night that I am definitely going to frame. In regard to me reaching for my goals, he wrote, "If they don't scare you, they are not *big* enough."

Throughout this Dave Ramsey financial boot camp, my husband and I have had *big* goals, and we are in it to achieve greatness together. Just like when I joined HIITBox, and the running burned my chest, and the sweat came out of my body like I'd unleashed the Hoover Dam, we will tackle our finances using the same concepts HIITBox taught me.

The Bible acknowledges hard work in Deuteronomy 15:10, saying, "God will bless you in all your work and in everything you put your hand to." **Like I told my trainer**, I have been given the tools to branch off and succeed in my workouts on my own during this season of paying off debt, and I have not worked this hard in my fitness goals to give up on myself again. But my tears still came that night! My heart still hurts because I never thought signing up for this financial class would be so life changing.

Another breakthrough I had was at the beginning of January 2018. I had started a *Beautifully Brave* journey with an online Bible study group. This journaling experience had me writing every day and challenging myself to be brave in areas I knew could use improvement. Since January, my prayer day after day was "God, please show me the ways to use my finances better and to be better prepared for unexpected expenses."

One day, my husband made the comment, "You only need me because I am the moneymaker." It was said during what I am sure was a kidding kind of moment, but for one reason or another, it stuck with me, and I wrote that down in my journal. Fast-forward to June 2018, and my husband was miserable at his day job. He was working too much—twelve-hour days, five days a week. Workers were unhappy at the job, so there was turnover galore in their warehouse. I was sure if my husband kept up with this schedule, soon he would be in the hospital, because I was sure he was going to give himself a heart attack. We agreed it was best for our family and for him if he quit his job. I stand by our mutual decision still to this day, and I am so proud of my husband for taking a stand for himself. Granted, we didn't think the unemployment would last five months and counting, but as a family, we have learned some valuable lessons as to who we are together and how we function. It is no coincidence we signed up for such a life-changing Financial Peace class through our church while we were living off of one income. Do you see, reader—all those times I prayed for clarity and prayed for a chance to be better at managing our finances, God was listening. Apparently I need to work on being "still" enough to hear him speak back, because it took this season of unemployment for my husband and I to finally get on the same page about our finances and our financial goals. This *big* picture all occurred to me in the same night, and I am not kidding when I say the tears just didn't stop!

What I am learning through this process is that it is completely okay to want *big* goals for yourself. It is also completely okay to admit you were wrong in your ways of thinking, and in my case, it was in my way of budgeting. Some may think talking about your financial problems shows the world your weaknesses, but think about it on the flip side; by sharing with the world that you were able to buy that house in cash or buy that new car in cash, how much more inspirational and motivational would that be to others who know you? I encourage you, think about those changes you want to make for yourself and your family, and write them down. If you believe in God, pray about it. What is standing in your way of turning those "wants" into actions? It's tough, you guys, and it might cause some tears, but it is so rewarding when you accomplish what your heart sets out to do.

I am so thankful to my family for encouraging me to just say the things I need to say. As a writer and someone who is writing a personal memoir, you wouldn't think telling your own story would be so hard. I am here to tell you, this was way harder than I thought, partly because my experiences and convictions are just what I said—personal. It is hard not to write a full paragraph saying all that you want to say then read it over and think, "Hmm, do I really want to tell the world all that?"

The thing that keeps me writing and keeps me from backing out of this whole book-writing process entirely is knowing in my heart that my story and experiences will resonate and help others. I hope to encourage readers to not hide their secrets but to share them. As I have learned, sharing such a personal testimony has only brought healing to the relationships closest to me. It has helped me to forgive myself and heal from the trauma of those hard situations. Writing this book has, to some extent, been intense therapy for me. I have been revived and felt some old memories just to allow myself to finally let go of the heartache. Writing this book has also had me sharing with my husband more about my childhood than I had ever shared with him or anyone else in my past. Backing my writing

Ch. 8 She is *Strong* for herself...

with scripture has also shown me that I am not the first person to experience such trials, nor will I be the last. Scripture already has us covered when it comes to crossroads in our lives. Big or small crossroads, scripture talks about them all, from love, forgiveness, happiness, sadness, life, death, and so much more. Isn't that inspiring? I've allowed myself to be my own worst critic all these years, but God, and what scripture has to say, already had me covered. I am writing to encourage you to be strong and say what you need to say.

CHAPTER 9
She is *Strong* but not finished . . .

Growing up, I always wanted to be a successful writer and photographer who traveled the world, took photos, and shared my stories with the world. It is crazy to me that I steered away from this dream to the degree that I did. I'm not entirely sure when I stopped allowing myself to believe that I could truly be anything I set my mind to. It wasn't until I became a mother and started telling my own child to dream big and talk about all his life goals that I realized I'd stopped holding myself to such a high standard years ago.

My life has now come full circle; I do believe we are meant to each live out our life's calling—whether we see our destiny early or later in life is up to us. I knew my passions from a young age, but I was not at all ready to accept and use those passions for anything good or meaningful. I had so much growing to do before I made it to where I am today. My mindset needed to be tested, my heart strengthened, and my body "still" to truly hear the answers to the many prayers I prayed. I strive to be obedient in this walk. I listen to the inner tugs at my heart that sometimes leave me feeling uncomfortable. My life experiences are hard to read and sometimes hard to process.

I write to show my readers I am not at all perfect; if anything, I would say I am still very much a work in progress in all areas of my life. A lot of what I have shared are things I have personally had to work through. I have never been to formal therapy for myself, not because I don't believe it could work for me, but because for so long I could hold in such trauma, such heartache, and remain a functioning member of society. Little did I know, God was equipping me for the hardest journey of them all, and that would be to share my personal testimony with you all. It is so true, the saying, "The truth will set you free." I have prayed over and over for God to show me the truth of who I really am. I was adamant in listening for the Lord's answer as to how such freedom was even possible. I wanted to be free from the lies I told myself and the lies I imagined others thought about me. I begged to be rescued! I wrote the words, "Bring me truth like a waterfall."

My story is not finished, and I am a work in progress—with God's help, sharing my truths with close friends, my husband, my family, and now with the world has finally set me free. I still practice daily what it means to give my worries to God. I take comfort in knowing I am not a mistake, and my mistakes are not what define me, and my past is not what defines me either. I am confident I have been given such hardships in my life because without those hardships and realities, I know within my core I would have been too stubborn to notice God's love on my own. The Bible says there is a part of me and a part of you that was made in God's image (Genesis 1:27). I would like to think one day I will have that conversation and get to ask, "Was it my strength that made me like you? What part of me was it that made me more like you?" Can you visualize such a conversation? Isn't that an incredible concept? I find it fascinating that our Bible is written by a bunch of sinners—a group of people like you and me who were chosen by God to share the word of God. Don't believe me? Open your Bible and start reading.

Ch. 9 She is *Strong* but not finished…

David committed murder and adultery. Paul persecuted and killed Christians, and the famous Moses was also a murderer.

There is a sense of freedom when you don't allow yourself to keep those skeletons in the closet any longer. I wouldn't have been able to write my first book had this been my decision alone. I am confident I am made for more, and in this season of personal development and growth, it is no coincidence God has me wanting to share my story with the world, even if to me it seems unfinished. Thank you, Lord, for entrusting me with such a task, knowing I too would be brave even when it came to sharing the hard stuff.

ABOUT THE AUTHOR

Victoria McCune is a passionate blogger who will write about almost anything, from the uncertainties of life to the beauty of confidence. She is honest about who she is and why her faith is so important to her. Victoria, who has served as a caregiver for most of her life, realized she could reach for more personal success and still care for those who need her most. Victoria comes from a rather large family, but in times of sickness and struggle, she has been inclined to seek help from only a few loved ones because she prefers to live life focused on others rather than herself. Victoria's passion to help people and encourage them not only surfaces in her writing but also through the way she lives her everyday life. Victoria lives out her passion as an active volunteer in her community, in her online Bible study group, and in her career as a financial counselor.